Forthcoming titles

Acupuncture in Clinical Practice

A guide for health professionals

Nadia Ellis MSc MCSP

Senior Physiotherapist, Stoke Mandeville Hospital,
Aylesbury, UK

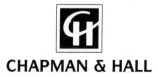

CHAPMAN & HALL

London · Glasgow · Weinheim · New York · Tokyo · Melbourne · Madras

Published by Chapman & Hall, 2–6 Boundary Row, London SE1 8HN, UK

Chapman & Hall, 2–6 Boundary Row, London SE1 8HN, UK

Blackie Academic & Professional, Wester Cleddens Road, Bishopbriggs, Glasgow G64 2NZ, UK

Chapman & Hall GmbH, Pappelallee 3, 69469 Weinheim, Germany

Chapman & Hall Inc., One Penn Plaza, 41st Floor, New York NY 10119, USA

Chapman & Hall Japan, Thomson Publishing Japan, Hirakawacho Nemoto Building, 6F, 1-7-11 Hirakawa-cho, Chiyoda-ku, Tokyo 102, Japan

Chapman & Hall Australia, Thomas Nelson Australia, 102 Dodds Street, South Melbourne, Victoria 3205, Australia

Chapman & Hall India, R. Seshadri, 32 Second Main Road, CIT East, Madras 600 035, India

Distributed in the USA and Canada by Singular Publishing Group Inc., 4284 41st Street, San Diego, California 92105

First edition 1994

© 1994 Nadia Ellis

Typeset in 10/12 pt Palatino by Best-set Typesetter Ltd, Hong Kong
Printed in Great Britain by St Edmundsbury Press, Bury St Edmunds, Suffolk

ISBN   0 412 47880 3   1 56593 179 3 (USA)

A catalogue record for this book is available from the British Library

Library of Congress Catalog Card Number 93-74440

∞ Printed on permanent acid-free text paper, manufactured in accordance with ANSI/NISO Z39.48-1992 and ANSI/NISO Z39.48-1984 (Permanence of Paper).

For
David, Stephen and Libba

Contents

Preface

My interest in acupuncture was first aroused while I was still at school and for a short period studied Mandarin. This enthusiasm came about from contact with a delegation of Chinese students at an International Arts festival where I was struck by the differences in our culture and lifestyle.

My schoolgirl ambition was to qualify as a physiotherapist and then go to Beijing to study acupuncture. The former was duly realized on leaving school; the latter was only partially fulfilled 18 years later when I enrolled in a Traditional Chinese Medicine course at the British College of Acupuncture in London. I have since then attended acupuncture courses in Nanjing and Guangzhou.

As a physiotherapist there are some areas of internal medicine that do not come under the remit of my clinical practice and this book is written for those practitioners who are primarily concerned in physical rehabilitation. It can be used not only as a reference book for those who are undertaking a training in acupuncture, but for all such as myself who are trained in Western medicine, but who wish to include traditional Chinese concepts of examination and diagnosis into their clinical practice.

Introduction

Acupuncture is now being included in the scope of physiotherapy practice in many parts of the world. This book is intended to give knowledge of both the Western and traditional Chinese concepts of acupuncture.

The section on traditional Chinese medicine (TCM) is only an outline of this vast subject but is somewhat longer than that devoted to Western medicine (WM) of which it is assumed that the reader will have basic knowledge. The intention is to give enough information to understand the reasoning behind the use of acupoints in treating different disorders encountered in clinical practice.

In order to be able to examine and treat a patient using the principles of TCM, the practitioner needs to have an awareness of the essential concepts of health and disease and an understanding of how energy or *qi* (*chi*, *ch'i*) can be manipulated using acupuncture techniques.

Methods of traditional examination are described and some practitioners will find them useful in obtaining a fuller picture of the problem presented. Others may not find these techniques appropriate in their practice, but the basic knowledge gained from Part One should help in their understanding of the foundations of acupuncture and enable them to use recommended acupoints with more knowledge of what energic changes are likely to occur.

There will be various techniques of non-invasive acupuncture described which will be useful to those practitioners who are not able as yet to pierce skin.

The final section of this book will include actual case histories, illustrating the combination of treatment that can be used in conditions that are met in clinical practice.

Part One

The Basic Concepts of Traditional Chinese Medicine (TCM)

1

The history of traditional Chinese medicine

The existence of traditional Chinese medicine (TCM) can be traced through written scripts as far back as 3000 years. One of the earliest text books on the subject is the *Huang Ti Nei Ching* or *The Yellow Emperor's Manual of Corporeal Medicine*. The first part called the *Su Wen* is written in a question and answer format between the legendary Emperor Huang Ti and his minister Chi-Po. This book can be dated back to the 2nd century BC although the practice of acupuncture and moxabustion is believed to be much older. Moxabustion is the name given to heat which is applied to the skin by burning the dried leaves of the herb *Artemisia vulgaris* (mugwort). Acupuncture and moxabustion are of equal importance in TCM and it is believed that moxabustion predated acupuncture as a treatment.

TCM is founded upon the holistic concept of treatment, and an acknowledgment of the body's ability to return to its balanced state of health, given the correct stimulus to do so. The two forces that need to be in balance are *yin* (negative) and *yang* (positive). These two energies are the opposing forces which govern the universe. Treatment is therefore undertaken bearing in mind the cause of the imbalance which manifests itself in symptoms, rather than addressing the symptoms primarily and leaving cause unrectified. It takes into account that the body is a self-repairing mechanism and any interference should be aimed at encouraging this self-healing ability. It is important to remember that 3000+ years ago there were no X-rays or laboratory tests that could be used to examine blood and other body substances. The doctor at that time had to rely on observation of the surface of the body, its temperature, colour of tongue, the pulses and the colour of the body waste, be it sputum, faeces or urine. To add to these observations, the cycles of the years, seasons, the change from night to day and the monthly phases of the moon, all had significance in discovering the nature of any disorder. An elaborate structure was formed to correlate all these natural phenomena into the theory of the Five Elements. These were identified as Fire, Earth, Metal, Water and Wood.

Although the concept of TCM springs from a completely different conceptual framework to that of Western medicine the *Su Wen*, which was compiled in the 2nd century BC, described blood continuously circulating in special transporting vessels. It was 1700 years later that Western medicine came round to this point of view.

The Chinese not only hypothesized on the circulation of blood but had worked out that it was pumped around the body by the heart and the rate and strength of this pump could be felt at the wrist. This led to the taking of pulses as a diagnostic examination procedure. It was also believed that there was another form of circulation in the body, that of *qi* (*chi, ch'i*). This had a *yin* and *yang* content mirroring the existence of the *yin* and *yang* energy of which the universe was composed.

The *qi* circulated in 12 channels of energy each governed by an organ. It is interesting to note that the brain was not considered to be a major organ, but merely a storage organ; the liver was believed to be the centre of intelligence and thought.

At certain points along these channels/meridians where they lay near the surface of the skin, small areas were identified which gave access to the channel. These areas were called acupoints. Acupuncture needles (the original ones being carved from stone) were inserted into these designated areas to release perverse influences from the interior of the body and restore balance.

A famous physician, San Su Mo, who lived between AD 581 and 673, devised a very clever method of locating acupoints. He recognized that his patients came in different shapes and sizes and to use a standard measurement for all of them was not logical. He used the distance between the creases of the distal and middle phalangeal folds when the patient's index finger was flexed, as a measure. This solved the difference in body structure and a simple length of straw or paper was cut to the correct length to act as a template for measuring on the patient the location of the acupoints. This modular 'inch' was called a *cun* or *pouce*.

Acupuncture was taught in the Imperial Medical College which was founded in the 1st century AD and soon there were colleges in every province of China. Examination of the medical students was rigorous. In their final examinations a bronze figure with holes to mark the acupoints was first filled with water and then sealed with wax and covered with rice paper. The student was asked to identify acupoints and place the needles in them. If they failed to locate the correct spot they missed the wax plug, there was no release of water and the student was failed.

The practice of TCM thrived until the 16th Century AD and then slowly declined mainly because there was an increasing number of missionaries from the West who brought with them Western concepts of medicine along with their religious beliefs. Western medical schools were increasingly taking over from the traditional Chinese medical colleges and acupuncture was relegated to the countryside and became the poor man's medicine.

It had a remarkable revival after the Second World War, when the new revolutionary government in China actively encouraged its rebirth. In the following chapters an outline of the basic theory of TCM will be given. The principles described will then be used to discuss how a patient can be examined, diagnosed and a treatment plan worked out.

2

The basis of traditional Chinese medicine

2.1 *YIN* AND *YANG*

The concept of *yin* and *yang* is that all matter consists of both negative and positive components. It is based on the philosophy of Tao. The essential nature of Tao was described in the 5th Century BC by Laotse in the Tao te king. The Tao is an abstract force that creates all things and brings about the polarity between *yin* and *yang* from an unstructured primal state. All things in nature develop within this field of tension between *yin* and *yang*. Examples of *yin* and *yang* are listed in Table 2.1.

In the living body *yin* and *yang* energies form the basis for illness and health. When *yin* and *yang* are in balance the body is in a state of good health (Figure 2.1a). The wavy line between the dark and light area indicates a constant movement between the two energies and the small contrasting areas in each indicate that within each energy mass there is the opposite. When there is too

Table 2.1 Examples of *yin* and *yang*

Yin	Yang
Female	Male
Dark	Light
Soft	Hard
Winter	Summer
Earth	Sky
Day	Night
Cold	Hot
Fat	Muscle
Solid	Hollow
Deep	Superficial

much *yang* this could indicate a 'hot' fever (Figure 2.1b). Or there could be an excess of *yin*, a deep 'cold' condition (Figure 2.1c), or no *yin* or *yang* energy (Figure 2.1d); this is clinical death.

It is clear that if something is overheated it needs to be cooled down and, using the same principle of balancing, a body that is too cold needs to be heated to restore health. Thus the principle of *yin* and *yang* forms an important part of diagnosis.

Yin and *yang* energy not only affects the body as a whole but at every level down to the cellular structure. Various outward manifestations can be identified, which give a guide to how the energy is balanced both in the body as a whole and in the various organs. The concept of *yin* and *yang* is just one aspect which is used in

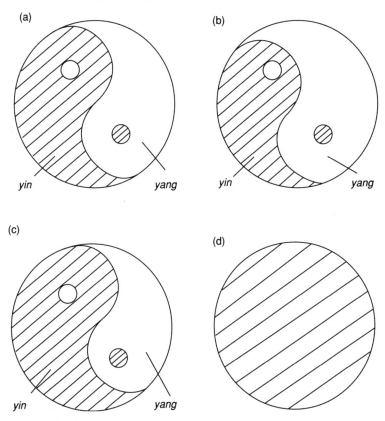

Figure 2.1 The Tao symbol for *yin* and *yang*: (a) a healthy balance, (b) excess of *yang* (deficiency of *yin*), (c) excess of *yin* (deficiency of yang), (d) clinical death.

Chinese diagnosis but forms the basis of the interpretation of disorders which are met in clinical practice.

2.2 VITAL ENERGY OR *QI*

This is sometimes written as chi or ch'i. Throughout this book 'qi' will be used.

Qi is the omnipresent force in all life. It manifests in the viscera, skin and permeates every living tissue. It accumulates in the organs and flows in the channels or meridians. It is described in various forms and densities in the living body.

2.2.1 *Hsien chien qi*

This is the ancestral form. It is divided into two parts

- *Ching qi*: which is stored in the kidney.
- *Yuan qi*: which derives from *ching qi* and circulates through the body.

It is derived from the combined *hsien chien qi* of the sperm and ovum when the fetus is formed and it cannot be replenished. Throughout life it is gradually used up and finally it is exhausted (clinical death).

2.2.2 *Hou t'ien qi*

This is acquired from air, food, etc. and is divided into five forms:

1. *Ku qi* derived from food and drink. This is described as intermediate energy and together with *t'ai qi* from the air it forms *zong qi* in the lungs.
2. *Zong qi* has two functions:
   a. It nourishes the heart and lung – respiration.
   b. Together with *yuan qi* it circulates in the meridians in its new form *chen qi*.
3. *Chen qi* is the energy circulating in the meridians and gives rise to *ying qi* (yin) and *wei qi* (yang).
4. *Ying qi* flows with blood and it is this energy that keeps the blood in its vessels. Therefore low *ying qi* could result in haemorrhage. It also nourishes the *zang* organs, which are the heart, pericardium, spleen, lung, kidney and liver.
5. *Wei qi*: this is defensive energy. It warms and nourishes tissues and organs, adjusts the opening and closing of pores, regulates

temperature and prevents the invasion of the external climatic perverse influences by concentrating at the surface of the body.

2.2.3 Conclusions

There is a deep circulation of energy uniting the inner organs and a superficial system which flows below the surface of the skin. The more superficial energy can be influenced from specific points on the surface of the skin. The deeper energy is not directly accessible, but can be influenced indirectly by surface points having the appropriate links.

The balance of *qi* in the various vital organs is important to health. When there is excess or deficiency there is malfunction, which gives rise to various illnesses.

The essence of diagnosis of any condition in traditional Chinese medicine is an assessment of the energy levels in the various systems described above. The means by which *qi* in the body is assessed is through the surface appearance of the individual and through various diagnostic procedures, e.g. examination of pulses and tongue, which will be discussed in later chapters.

2.3 THE FIVE ELEMENTS

The essence of this ancient tradition is that *yin* and *yang*, in addition to exerting their dual power, are subdivided in to the Five Elements: Fire, Earth, Metal, Water and Wood. Man, who is said to be the product of heaven and earth by the interaction of *yin* and *yang*, also contains the five elements. This close relationship between the Five Elements and the human body is expressed in the Five Element Correspondences.

2.3.1 The *sheng* cycle (Figure 2.2)

The Five Elements are conceived as being organized into a cycle of energy thus:

Metal creates Water;
Water creates Wood;
Wood creates Fire;
Fire creates Earth;
Earth creates Metal.

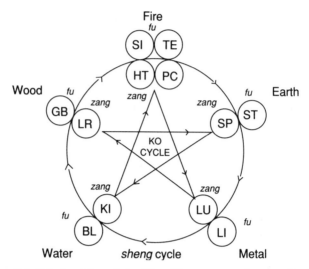

Figure 2.2 Relationship of the Five Elements to the *zang/fu* organs, showing the *sheng* cycle.

Each element has an association with the organs of the body: lung (LU), large intestine (LI), stomach (ST), spleen (SP), heart (HT), small intestine (SI), bladder (BL), kidney (KI), pericardium (PC), triple energizer (TE), gall bladder (GB) and liver (LR). Energy passes clockwise through the elements to form the *sheng* cycle. There are other correspondences associated with the elements: the seasons, external climatic conditions, the emotions (Figure 2.3); body tissues, five senses, tastes, body fluids and functions (Figure 2.4). Disorders can be looked at taking into account the various factors which are described in the Five Element Theory. Consideration of both the emotional and physical factors is an important part of traditional diagnosis.

2.3.2 Metal

The colour is white. The season is autumn and the organs lung (*zang*) and large intestine (*fu*). The associated tissue is skin and mucous membrane. The nose and sense of smell are associated with mucous membrane. The climatic influence is dryness. The tasts is sour and the internal emotion grief.

For example, asthma, a respiratory disease involving the

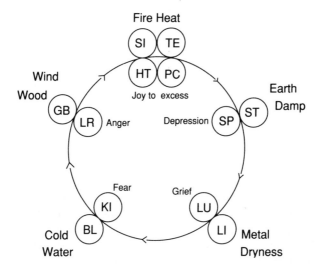

Figure 2.3 Relationship of the Five Elements to internal emotions and external influences.

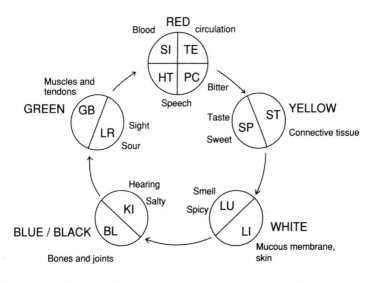

Figure 2.4 The Five Element Correspondences showing the associated colours, body tissues and senses.

smooth muscle of the bronchioles of the lungs, can be accompanied by eczema, a dry and irritating skin condition.

When taking a history the patient who is grieving, for whatever reason, may be exhibiting disturbances in the lung and large intestine, crying a great deal, or suffering with various skin problems.

2.3.3 Water

The colour is blue/black. The season is winter, the external climatic influence is cold, the organs kidney (*zang*) and bladder (*fu*), the tissue is bone. The sense of hearing and the ear are associated with this element. The taste is salty and the internal emotion fear. For example, a disturbance in this element could affect the joints and bones as in osteoarthritis. There can also be some urinary disturbances. It is sometimes found in an elderly person suffering from osteoarthritis that they also have nocturia. Treating the local joint pain and the Water element systemically with acupuncture may affect nocturia.

When the body ages the stored Ancestral Energy (*yuan qi*) in the kidneys declines and it is often the case that elderly people have impaired hearing.

Dark (blue/black) shadows under the eyes will often denote a kidney disturbance especially after a night of excessive alcohol intake which has a dehydrating effect on the system.

The emotion of grief should not be ignored in assessing the influence of this element on a presenting condition.

2.3.4 Wood

The colour is green. The season is spring, the climatic influence Wind, the organs liver (*zang*) and gall bladder (*fu*), the tissue is muscle, the internal emotion anger and the taste sour. The eyes and vision are influenced by this element.

For example, it is not uncommon to develop a stiff neck when travelling in a car with a window open, causing a draught on the back of the head and neck. This would be described as an invasion of Wind and gall bladder acupoints in the area would be used to expel the Wind.

A greenish complexion can also be the result of any liver disease and anger is often described as 'rising gall'.

2.3.5 Fire

The colour is red. The season is summer, the external influence heat, the organs are the heart, pericardium (*zang*), small intestine and triple energizer (*fu*). The function is the circulation which includes blood vessels and blood. The climatic influence is heat. The tongue and associated speech come into this element.

For example, high fever and excessive thirst and haemoptysis are symptoms which can be demonstrated as well as heart problems such as myocardial infarct and angina. Heart conditions are accompanied by a florid complexion and sufferers do not like hot weather. The internal emotion is joy to excess or mania. An important piece of advice given to those who have a 'heart condition' is not to get over-excited or stressed.

2.3.6 Earth

The colour is yellow/brown. The season is late summer, the climatic influence damp, the organs are spleen (*zang*) and stomach (*fu*) and the tissue is connective tissue. The sense of taste and tongue come under this element. The taste is sweetness and the internal emotion is depression.

For example, it is often the case that when feeling depressed one turns to sweets and chocolates. This increases the depression and a damaging cycle can be set up. In dealing with many patients the physiotherapist is likely to encounter a musculo-skeletal condition accompanied by some degree of depression. It is surprising how many are addicted to sweet tasting foods. The antidote could be to advise them to stop eating the sweet things and start eating savoury or sour foods.

The patient who complains of heaviness in the limbs and dull aching joints could be suffering from insufficient SP *qi* causing Phlegm (Damp). This is Internal Damp.

Stomach and spleen syndromes are often accompanied by a brownish colour of the skin and are exacerbated in damp weather.

2.3.7 The *ko* cycle (Figure 2.2)

This has a controlling influence over the organs. Thus:

Water controls Fire;
Fire controls Metal;

Metal controls Wood;
Wood controls Earth;
Earth controls Water.

It can be seen that imbalance in the *zang/fu* can be caused not only by problems in the *sheng* cycle but also in the *ko* cycle.

For example, the heart is nourished by the liver which is its mother or controlled by the kidney across the *ko* cycle.

If there is a 'full' heart condition it could be the result of a lack of control from the kidney, which is weak. If the heart is weak (*xu*) it could be due to lack of *qi* coming from the liver (the mother) or an over-strong kidney, which is overcoming the *qi* in the heart across the *ko* cycle.

2.3.8 Perverse energy

Symptoms presented can often give a clue as to which of the perverse energies of the Five Elements is causing the problem.

(a) Wind (Fong)

External
This is shifting pain attacking the upper part of the body. Traditional point of entry is GV 16 (*fengfu*) travelling to GB 20 (*fengchi*), which will give occipital pain and headache. It then descends to GV 14 (*dazhui*) and causes shoulder pain. The further superficial penetration into the tendino-muscular meridians will cause coughs, blocked eyes and sneezing. If *wei qi* is insufficient to counteract the invasion there will be penetration to the main meridians causing fever with perspiration and severe headaches. The tongue will have a white fur covering.

Internal
This can cause dysfunction of the liver and disturbances of the circulation to the upper part of the body. 'Uprising wind' can cause an excess of *yang qi* in the liver. The resulting symptoms could be dizziness, tinnitus, muscle spasms, deviation of mouth or eyes (Bell's palsy) and numbness of the extremities.

It is interesting to note that traditional texts point out that if a tongue is deviated and cannot be kept still when protruded, it signifies that there is a deep invasion of Wind and a stroke (cerebral thrombosis) may follow. Treatment would involve sedating liver *yang* by needling LR 2 (*xingjian*), which is the Fire point, at the same time tonifying liver *yin* by treating LR 3 (*taichong*) which is the *yuan* (source) point.

Empty blood wind

This describes wind attacking blood. Symptoms will include: Shaking, vertigo, headaches, floaters in the eyes, stiffness of the spine and/or low back pain. Tongue: pale. Pulses: fine and choppy.

Hot blood wind

This is more common in elderly people. It is characterized by: Sudden onset of violent headaches, tinnitus, vertigo, and hypertension. Tongue: dark red, deviated and quivering. Pulses: wiry and full.

In this case treatment would aim to eliminate Wind GV 14 (*dazhui*) and cool the blood LI 4 (*hegu*), LR 3 (*taichong*).

(b) Heat (Shu)

Perverse heat tends to exhaust body *qi*. This results in dehydration. Symptoms include: Thirst, fever, headache, dry mouth. Tongue: thick white fur and looks greasy. Pulses: full and fluctuating.

(c) Humidity (Shih)

This is likely to invade the body in late summer when the weather is more inclined to be damp and humid.

It is often associated with other perverse energies to produce Damp/Heat, or Damp/Cold.

The resulting condition is a block to the smooth flow of *qi*. Symptoms include: Purulent discharges, severe headache, abdominal distension, aching joints and yellow sclera. Tongue: smooth, greasy, with yellow fur. Pulses: feel soft.

(d) Dryness (Zao)

This is rare. It can occur when there is no rain in late summer. This would mean that the lungs have been deprived of moist air prior to the dry autumn when *qi* is at its fullest in the Metal element. Symptoms include: Dry cough, energy rising to the head, pain in the lungs.

(e) Cold (Han)

Superficial
Attacks peripheral blood vessels and *wei qi*. This results in the inhibition of blood *qi* circulation. Symptoms include: Headache, fever, lack of perspiration, dislike of cold and general aches and pains. Tongue: pale with white fur. Pulses: superficial and hard.

Deep
Painful joints; cold increases and heat relieves pain. This is quite often demonstrated in clinical practice. Some patients get relief of pain with application of ice, others when heat is given.

Penetration to the ST and SP organs causes vomiting of clear fluid, diarrhoea and abdominal pain. This leads further to increased internal *yin*. There will be extreme pallor and coldness of arms and legs. Pulses: deep and submerged.

(f) Fire (Huo)

This is not the external climatic perverse energy of Fire but internally generated fire. Symptoms include: Very severe fever, flushed face, congested, concentrated urine, and extreme thirst. Tongue: red with yellow fur. Pulses: rapid. *Huo* combines with other internal perverse energies to produce internal fire. Symptoms include: Haemorrhage, haemoptysis and extreme anger. If the TE is affected it can result in tonsillitis and halitosis.

2.3.9 Delayed symptoms

There is the phenomenon of delayed reaction to external climatic influences, which can further complicate diagnosis.

Invasion of *fong* in the spring can cause diarrhoea in the summer. Invasion of *shu* in the summer can cause intermittent fever in the autumn.

Invasion of *shih* in the autumn can cause cough in the winter. Invasion of *han* in the winter can produce superficial *yang* disturbances in the spring.

2.3.10 Conclusions

The acceptance of the theory of the Five Elements is difficult for one trained in Western concepts of medicine. In the author's experience the awareness of Five Element Theory has been very helpful in taking a history even when acupuncture is not the treatment of choice. Signs and symptoms which appear unrelated in Western concepts of medicine can usually be understood using Five Element Theory.

In the United States there is some activity to investigate the Five Element Theory, relating this to developing a mathematical model for acupuncture meridians (Friedman *et al.*, 1989).

When taking a case history, the date of birth may have some significance in the patient's presenting problem. The time of day, the year of birth and the month can all be correlated using Five Element Theory.

The above is only a summary of a wealth of information which has accumulated over thousands of years. It gives a different and fascinating aspect to the diagnosis of disorders which are met in clinical practice.

2.4 THE EIGHT PRINCIPLES OF DIAGNOSIS

In traditional Chinese medicine, the correlation of signs and symptoms are classified into eight main categories. There are various examination procedures which enable the practitioner to arive at a diagnosis based on the Eight Principles. This includes pulse and tongue examination. The technique of pulse taking and tongue diagnosis is addressed in Chapter 3. The Eight Principles of diagnosis are described below:

1. Internal/external
2. Hot/cold
3. Full/empty
4. *Yin/yang*

2.4.1 Internal/external

(a) Internal disturbances (Li)

These are disharmonious states of the *zang* and *fu* organs.

When combined with an invasion of **Cold** the symptoms are characterized by abdominal and thoracic pain and there is fear of cold. Pulse: floating and slow. Tongue: lightly coloured with a thick coating.

When combined with an invasion of **Heat** there is dryness of the mouth, thirst and restlessness. Pulse: rapid and very full. Tongue: feels tender, appears thick and has a white coating.

When combined with **Emptiness** the limbs feel cold. There is dizziness, fatigue, diarrhoea and palpitations. Pulse: deep and weak. Tongue: thick, tender, whitish coating.

When combined with **Fullness** there may be halitosis, lack of perspiration of hands and feet. There is a feeling of pressure in the chest. Pulse: deep and full. Tongue: has a yellow coat and is dry.

(b) External problems (Biao)

These are, as expected, to do with superficial disturbances and influenced by climate such as cold, heat, damp or wind. Complaints in this category would include neuralgia and localized joint disease.

When combined with **Cold** there is fever and shivering. Pulse: floating and light. Tongue: has a white coating.

When combined with **Heat** there is a hot skin and thirst. Pulse: rapid and floating. Tongue: thin white coating with a red tip.

When combined with an **Empty** condition, there is perspiration and a feeling of cold. Pulse: weak, floating and slow. Tongue: pale.

When combined with a **Full** condition, there is general pain and a lack of perspiration. Pulse: floating, rapid, strong. Tongue: white coating.

2.4.2 Hot/cold

(a) Hot conditions (Re)

These are caused by increased *yang* activity of the *qi* in the body. Heat is generated and *yin* energy is overcome, the result being a high temperature, hyperaemia, pain and agitation. The symptoms experienced would be: lack of saliva, yellow thick sputum, constipation, likes to stretch, warm limbs, reddish complexion, lips swollen, likes cold drinks. Pulse: floating, over-full, rapid, strong. Tongue: coarse coating which is dry and yellow or dry and black. The body of the tongue appears shrivelled and tough.

(b) Cold conditions (Han)

These occur when external pathogenic cold affects the body more deeply. This gives rise to chronic conditions, the *yang* energy being overwhelmed. The symptoms experienced would be: Excess of saliva, sputum thick and white, diarrhoea, likes to huddle, cold limbs, pale complexion and lips, likes hot drinks. Pulse: deep, fine, slow and weak. Tongue: moist, tender, with no coating or with a thin white coat.

2.4.3 Full/empty

(a) Full conditions (Shi)

These are signified by an excess of *qi* and the symptoms give rise to acute cramps, hypertension, increased muscle tone. Psychological restlessness, e.g. agitation and insomnia, is one of the symptoms encountered. Pulse: overflowing, slippery and strong. Tongue: tough, thick coating.

(b) Empty conditions (Xu)

These are caused by deficiency of *qi*. This leads to hypofunction of the organs and typical symptoms will be excessive tiredness, exhaustion, low blood pressure, tinnitus, incontinence of urine, diarrhoea and sudden profuse sweating.

The diseases are usually chronic and the result of the draining of *qi* over a long period. Pulse: very small, fine and weak. Tongue: light coloured with a thin coating.

2.4.4 *Yin* and *yang*

These are the categories within Chinese thought that have universal validity and are applicable to all phenomena. The diagnosis criteria described above – interior/exterior, excess/deficiency, heat/cold – should be regarded as shadings of the overall concept of *yin* and *yang*. Thus for example, excess and heat are *yang* criteria and internal and cold are *yin* criteria. Looking at the tongue and pulse can be an important guide to the dominance of a *yin* or *yang* condition.

(a) Yang

Pulse: floating, overflowing, rapid, slippery, full and strong. Tongue: the body will be red, shrivelled, and tough; the coating yellow with cracks or blackish with pimples.

(b) Yin

Pulse: deep, minute, fine, rough, slow, empty and weak. Tongue: body light coloured, thick and tender; coating appears glossy.

2.4.5 Conclusions

Having learned all the various aspects of signs and changes in tongue and pulse, etc. there comes a time when this has to be correlated with the presenting symptoms.

It is not easy to combine TCM and Western concepts of diagnosis. It is easier to practise solely in one or other discipline.

The physiotherapist is primarily trained to fulfil the function of treating patients in a physical way and is probably working with a patient who is also attending a medical practitioner. In these circumstances one cannot ignore the Western diagnosis or the medication that has possibly been prescribed. However, this need not interfere with the successful management of symptoms for which the patient has been referred. Indeed, knowledge of the Eight Principles of diagnosis can enable the physiotherapist to treat not only the symptoms which are presented, but also the underlying cause of those symptoms.

2.5 THE SIX *CHIAOS*

2.5.1 Introduction

This is the concept of describing layers of energy, using the knowledge of the Eight Principles of Diagnosis, Meridian Theory and Five Element Correspondences (Figure 2.5).

Perverse energy penetrates the body from the surface and the health and balance of the individual become further compromised as the perverse energy penetrates to the deeper energy layers. The theory of the Six *Chiaos* is very complex and only a simple outline will be given in this chapter.

The Six *Chiaos* are conceptual concentric protective layers which defend the vital inner organs. They are described from the most superficial defensive layer below:

External: SI and BL *tai yang* or great *yang*
           TE and GB *chao yang* or lesser *yang*
   to   LI and ST *yang ming* or bright *yang*
Internal: LU and SP *tai yin* or great *yin*
           PC and LR *tsui yin* or decreasing *yin*
           HT and KI *chao yin* or lesser *yin*

If the pairing of the Six *Chiaos* is examined with regard to the perverse elements involved, it will be noted that one balances out the other.

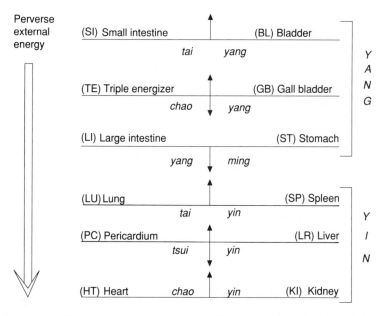

Figure 2.5 Diagrammatic representation of the Six *Chiaos*, showing their associated organs and relative exposure to perverse external energy.

Tai yang (SI/BL)	heat and cold
Chao yang (TE/GB)	heat and wind
Yang ming (LI/ST)	dryness and humidity
Tai yin (LU/SP)	dryness and humidity
Tsui yin (PC/LR)	heat and wind
Chao yin (HT/KI)	heat and cold

Each *chiao*, however, has its own predominant character. Thus:

Tai yang	cold
Chao yang	heat
Yang ming	dryness
Tai yin	humidity
Tsui yin	wind
Chao yin	fire

If, for example, *tai yang* is affected by cold, this can be countered by heat from *chao yin*. This could be done by using the transverse LO vessel (HT 5 *tongli*) from the heart to the small intestine and at the same time tonifying the energy in the heart by stimulating the *yuan* point (HT 7 *shenmen*) of the heart (Low, 1983).

2.5.2 Symptoms related to the Six *Chiaos*

(a) Tai yang

Subject can suffer invasion of:

1. Wind, causing fever, perspiration and fear of wind.
   Pulse: full and slow.
   Tongue: whitish fur.
2. Cold, causing fever, fear of cold and no perspiration.
   Pulse: full and strong.
   Tongue: whitish fur.
3. Heat, causing thirst and possible headaches.
   Pulse: full and rapid.
   Tongue: light red with white or yellow coating.

(b) Chao yang

This forms the hinge between the surface and deeper layers. If perverse energy penetrates to this level the symptoms will include: bouts of fever and shivering, pain over the heart with vomiting and a bitter taste in the mouth.

The involvement with GB and TH will produce pain in the throat, chest, sides and hips.

(c) Yang ming

When perverse energy has penetrated this level the colon and stomach will be affected as well as the meridians.

1. Affected meridians:
   Pulse: erratic and full.
   Tongue: red with white fur.

There will be copious sweating, thirst and anxiety.

2. Affected viscera:
   Pulse: deep, full and hard.
   Tongue: either yellow and moist or black and dry.

Pain in the stomach, constipation, abdominal distension, intermittent fever, perspiration and thirst.

(d) Tai yin

The symptoms are now of a *yin* nature with perverse cold affecting the spleen with humidity.
Pulse: slow weak pulse.
Tongue: heavy yellow coating.

(e) Tsui yin

This is the *yin* hinge, and *yin* and *yang* energy intermingle causing a variety of symptoms. These can be divided into four categories:

1. Heat of *yang* origin: causing painful diarrhoea.
2. Heat above and cold below: a feeling of energy rising in the chest, pain in the heart, vomiting after food and hunger but patient cannot eat.
3. Alternating heat and cold: causing fever and shivering. When *yang* is dominant the patient will recover, but when *yin* predominates the illness will continue.
4. Cold, due to 'emptiness in the blood': the limbs become cold and the pulses very weak.

(f) Chao yin

This is the deepest layer, housing the fire of the heart and the *yin* energy of the kidneys. Symptoms vary according to which energy, *yin* or *yang*, is involved.

Perverse cold affects the heart fire and results in emptiness of *yang*. Symptoms include: diarrhoea, vomiting, extreme fatigue and cold limbs. Pulses: thin and soft. Tongue: bright red with no coating.

When *yin* is compromised symptoms include: restlessness, pain in the heart area, pain in the chest and throat. Pulses: thin and soft. Tongue: red, no coating.

2.5.3 Conclusions

In clinical practice it is useful to have some concept of the layers of protective energy of the body. Knowledge of the symptoms in relation to the Six *Chiaos* should be kept in mind before reaching a diagnosis and deciding on a programme of treatment.

2.6 THE FOUR SEAS

In TCM the body is divided into three functional areas.

(1) Heaven: The area above the diaphragm including the lungs, heart and pericardium.
(2) Earth: Abdominal viscera including the spleen, stomach and gall bladder.
(3) Man: Includes the area below the umbilicus and includes the liver, kidney, intestine, bladder and uterus.

Controlling the balance of energy in 'Heaven, Earth and Man' are the Four Seas. These are:

1. Energy
2. Nourishment
3. Meridians/blood
4. Marrow

2.6.1 Sea of energy

The essence of the sea of energy is Heaven.

This sea controls the movement of energy derived from the air through respiration, into Earth and Man.

Acupoints with specific functions

- CV 17, *shanzhong*, is concerned with inspiring air.
- ST 9, *renying*, controls the ascent of *yang qi* from Man towards Heaven.
- BL 10, *tianzhu*, controls the descent of *yang* from Heaven to Earth and Man.

2.6.2 Sea of nourishment

The essence of this sea is Earth, where energy is extracted from food to nourish the whole body.

Acupoints with specific functions

- ST 30, *qichong*, controls the metabolism of *yang* nourishment and *qi* distribution.
- ST 36 *zusanli*, regulates the GB, SI, LI and BL, all digestion and drainage of the lower part of the body via Energy of Blood.

2.6.3 Sea of meridians/blood

The essence of this sea is the control of the interior of the body.

Acupoints with specific functions

- BL 11, *dashu*, binds the material aspect of bone and the immaterial aspect of the meridians.
- ST 37, *shangjuxu*, governs all movements from *yang* to *yin* as *summer* merges into *autumn*.
- ST 39, *xiajuxu*, governs all movements from *yin* to *yang* as winter merges into spring.

2.6.4 Sea of marrow

The essence of this sea is the control of the exterior. It governs all the means of contact with the exterior of limbs and head and acts like an antenna for the eyes, ears, nose and mouth.

Acupoints which are specific to the sea of marrow

GV 16 *fengfu* and GV 20 *bahui*.

The Four Seas can also be called the seas of heaven, earth, interior and exterior.

2.6.5 Symptomatology

Sea of energy.
Full: pain in chest, red face and dyspnoea.
Empty: Not enough energy to talk.

Sea of nourishment.
Full: abdominal distension.
Empty: anger with lack of appetite.

Sea of meridians/blood.
Full: body feels swollen or enlarged.
Empty: feels body is shrunk for no reason and feels resentment.

Sea of marrow.
Full: light sensations in the body, feelings of strength.
Empty: tinnitus, blurred vision, dizziness, fatigue of legs and desire to sleep.

Treatment incorporating the Four Seas should only be embarked on when other treatments have not been successful. The acupoints have a strong effect and should be needled using an 'even' technique. This is described in Chapter 5.

REFERENCES

Friedman M.J., Birch S. and Tiller, W.A. (1989) Towards the development of a mathematical model for acupuncture meridians. *Acupuncture and Electro-Therapeutics Res. Int. J.*, **14**, 217–226.

Low, R. (1983) Formation of Acupuncture Energies, in *The Secondary Vessels of Acupuncture*, Thorsons Publishers Ltd, Wellingborough, Northamptonshire.

FURTHER READING

Vieth, I. (1972) *The Yellow Emperor's Classic of Internal Medicine*, University of California Press, Berkeley, Los Angeles, London.

3

Meridian theory

3.1 INTRODUCTION

According to traditional Chinese medicine vital energy or *qi* flows through a system of 12 channels and regulates body functions. These channels are called meridians. Each meridian is identified with an organ or function. These paths of energy can be mapped on the surface of the body and specific points can be identified (acupoints) which, if pierced, can affect this flow of energy.

It is essential in the understanding of meridian theory to be familiar with the Five Element Correspondences which have been described in an earlier chapter and illustrated in Figure 2.4. The organs are divided into six pairs, which are the functional units. One organ in each pair being *yin* (*zang*) and one *yang* (*fu*). The meridians of the paired organs run parallel to one another and are connected at the periphery through the *lo* points. The *yang* meridians run laterally or on the dorsal side of the body, while the *yin* meridians run on the medial or ventral side. The 12 meridians together with the *lo* connections are collectively known as the *Jing-lo* System.

3.2 THE ORGANS

The six *fu* organs are stomach (ST), large intestine (LI), urinary bladder (BL), gall bladder (GB), small intestine (SI) and triple energizer (TE).

The six *zang* organs are spleen (SP), lung (LU), kidney (KI), liver (LR), heart (HT) and pericardium (PC).

Thus ST is paired with SP: Earth
       LI is paired with LU: Metal
       BL is paired with KI: Water

GB is paired with LR: Wood
SI is paired with HT: Fire
PC is paired with TE: Fire

3.2.1 The *zang* organs

Heart (*xin*) governs all other organs and regulates the flow of blood and *qi*. It stores and rules the mental energy, the mind and consciousness. The heart and pericardium form a functional unit, the latter organ being responsible for the circulation of blood and *qi*. The influencing climatic factor is Heat and the internal emotion is Joy to excess or agitation.

Lung (*fei*) controls the respiration and is responsible for the intake of *qi*. The lung governs the surface of the body, the skin and hair and has influence on the nose and mucous membrane. The climatic factor is Dryness and the internal emotion Grief.

Spleen (*pi*) controls the digestion of food and is responsible for the intake of fluids. It assimilates the *qi* from nutrition and nourishes and moves the blood. It governs the connective tissue and holds the organs in place. It opens to the mouth and is manifested in the lips. The external climatic influence is Dampness and the internal emotional influence is Depression.

Liver (*gan*) is responsible for the movement of body fluids. It controls the movements of the body and nourishes the muscles and tendons. It also nourishes the eyes. The external climatic influence is Wind and the internal emotional influence is Anger.

Kidney (*shen*) controls reproduction and is the organ where ancestral energy or *yuan qi* is stored. It eliminates impure fluids. It nourishes the bones, joints and teeth, rules the ears and manifests in head hair. The energy is depleted in old age, thus hair loses colour and thickness. Some elderly people have a reduced hearing capacity. The external climatic influence is Cold and the internal emotional influence Fear.

3.2.2 The *fu* organs

The function of these organs approximates the Western concepts of their function. However there is one which needs further examination.

The Triple Energizer

This organ does not exist as an entity but as a function. The Triple Energizer is brought into existence at the point when the umbilical cord is cut at parturition. The three energies it controls are:

Heaven (the Upper Energizer) which is described as that influencing the thorax and head controlling the area above the diaphragm. It is responsible for the assimilation of *qi* from the air through the lungs.
Earth (the Middle Energizer), the area below the diaphragm and above the pelvis. It is responsible for the digestion and absorption of useful foods, passing the waste into the large bowel for excretion.
Man (the Lower Energizer), the pelvic area which includes the sexual and excretory organs. It is an important contributory factor in both excretion of waste and in sexual function.

The existence of this fictional organ can possibly be related to the fact that in ancient times there was no systematic study of anatomy through post-mortem and the various functions of the body had to be explained by careful *in vivo* study. Thus two of the main 12 meridians, the Triple Energizer and the pericardium, do not have identifiable organs although they have identified meridian pathways and their functions form a vital part of good health.

In addition to the 12 coupled meridians there are the Extraordinary Channels, sometimes called the eight extra meridians. Two of these have their own identified channels.

Ren mai or Conception (CV) runs up the midline from the symphysis pubis to the mouth anteriorly. This is **yin** and is the centre of *yin* energy in the meridian system.

Du mai or Governor (GV), which is **yang** and is the centre of *yang* energy, runs up the midline of the spine, from the anus posteriorly over the head to the mouth, where it meets the Conception Meridian. These two meridians together with the 12 described earlier form the system of 14 channels on which the 361 classic acupuncture points are situated.

3.3 THE FLOW OF ENERGY

The Twelve Main Channels make up a continuous system for the flow of energy and can be described in three courses.

3.3.1 Course 1

Energy flows out of the LU and into the arm to the thumb. It then connects with the LI at the lateral nail point of the index finger and flows up the lateral aspect of the arm and neck to the side of the nose (LI 20 *yingxiang*).

It connects with the ST via BL 1 (*jingming*) and passes over the mandible and the temporo-mandibular joint to the hairline and emerges in the neck lateral to the trachea. It then follows an anterior course 4 cun lateral to the midline in the thorax and 2 cun from the midline in the abdomen. It then descends in an antero-lateral line down the leg and passes over the anterior aspect of the ankle into the foot to the lateral nail point of the second toe.

Then it connects with the SP which ascends from the medial nail point of the hallux, up the medial aspect of the leg and into the abdomen lateral to the ST meridian, ending on the lateral aspect of the chest. This completes the first course. The energy then passes into the HT.

3.3.2 Course 2

This starts with the energy entering the HT and flowing from the axilla down the antero-medial aspect of the arm and hand to the nail point of the little finger. It then connects with the SI ascending from the medial nail point of the little finger up the dorsal posterior aspect of the arm and shoulder to the maxilla. It then connects with the BL which passes from the canthus over the head, descending down the back lateral to the spinal column into the posterior aspect of the leg and lateral aspect of the foot to finish at the nail point of the little toe. It then connects with the KI meridian and ascends from the mid point of the transverse arch up the medial aspect of the leg and posterior to the SP, then into the medial aspect of the thigh and up into the abdomen medial to the stomach meridian to the second rib space. This completes the second course. The energy then enters the PC.

3.3.3 Course 3

The third course starts with the energy entering the PC, passing into the arm from the fourth rib space and descending to the lateral nail point of the third finger following the midline on the anterior aspect of the forearm. It then connects with the TE which ascends from the medial nail point of the third finger up the midline of the posterior aspect of the arm to the eyebrow.

The energy then passes into the GB and travels over the lateral aspect of the head from a point lateral to the eye, descending down the lateral aspect of the torso and side of the thigh and leg to the lateral nail point of the fourth toe.

The final link is to the LR which ascends from the lateral nail point of the hallux up the medial aspect of the leg and thigh, circles the genitalia and finishes in the seventh rib space. This completes the third course and the energy then enters the LU to begin the cycle all over again.

This flow of energy takes 24 hours allowing two hours per meridian. In traditional Chinese medicine *qi* enters the lung at 3.00 am and finishes in the liver at 3.00 am, 24 hours later (Figure 3.1).

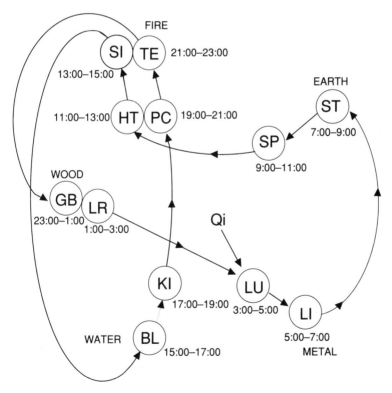

Figure 3.1 The circulation of *qi* through the meridian system showing the 24-hour cycle.

3.4 ENERGY CYCLES

There are two cycles which are important in assessing the level of energy in each of the meridians.

3.4.1 The seasonal cycle

The seasons are calculated according to the equinox dates on the calendar.

Thus summer starts on 21st June, autumn on 21st October, winter on 21st December and spring on 21st March. Late summer is considered to be the last month of the summer period. For example, stomach and spleen will be at their maximum influence and energy in late summer, the energy passing clockwise through the lung and large intestine (autumn), kidney and bladder (winter), liver and gall bladder (spring), small intestine, heart, triple energizer and pericardium (summer).

3.4.2 The 24-hour cycle

According to traditional Chinese theory, *qi* enters the lung at 3.00 am and circulates through the *zang/fu* system, taking 2 hours to pass through each organ, finishing in the liver between 1.00 and 3.00 am.

3.5 COMMAND POINTS

These can also be called 'Antique' or '*jing well*' points. The meridians flow near to the surface of the body in the lower limb up to the knee and in the upper limb to the elbow. They then move deeper into the tissues; therefore it is where the meridians are near to the surface that the command points are sited.

Five of the points relate to the five elements, the sixth to the source point (in the *fu* organs only) and the seventh to the paired organ, i.e. *lo* point.

Much of the work of balancing the pulses is done using these points. The principles only will be discussed in this section. Tables 3.1 and 3.2 show the command points of the *zang* and *fu* meridians while Table 3.3 shows the eight influential points.

Table 3.1 Command points *zang* organs

Meridians	Wood Jing-well	Fire Yung-spring	Earth Shu-stream	Metal Jing-river	Water He-sea/ho	Lo	Yuan
(LU) Lung	LU 11 *shaoshang*	LU 10 *yuji*	LU 9 *taiyuan*	LU 8 *jingqu*	LU 5 *chize*	LU 7 *lieque*	LU 9 *taiyuan*
(SP) Spleen	SP 1 *yinbai*	SP 2 *dadu*	SP 3 *taibai*	SP 5 *shangqiu*	SP 9 *yinlinguan*	SP 4 *gongsun*	SP 3 *taibai*
(HT) Heart	HT 9 *shaochong*	HT 8 *shaofu*	HT 7 *shenmen*	HT 4 *lingdao*	HT 3 *shaohai*	HT 5 *tongli*	HT 7 *shenmen*
(KI) Kidney	KI 1 *yongquan*	KI 2 *rangu*	KI 3 *taixi*	KI 7 *fuliu*	KI 10 *shaohai*	KI 4 *dazhong*	KI 3 *taixi*
(PC) Pericardium	PC 9 *zhongchong*	PC 8 *laogong*	PC 7 *daling*	PC 5 *jianshi*	PC 3 *quze*	PC 6 *neiguan*	PC 7 *daling*
(LR) Liver	LR 1 *dadun*	LR 2 *xingjian*	LR 3 *taichong*	LR 4 *zhongfeng*	LR 8 *ququan*	LR 5 *ligou*	LR 3 *taichong*

Table 3.2 Command points *fu* organs

Meridians	Metal jing-well	Water yung-spring	Wood shu-stream	Fire jing-river	Earth he-sea/ho	Lo	Yuan
(LI) Large intestine	LI 1 shangyang	LI 2 erjian	LI 3 sanjian	LI 5 yangxi	LI 11 quchi	LI 6 pianli	LI 4 hegu
(ST) Stomach	ST 45 lidui	ST 44 neiting	ST 43 xiangu	ST 41 jiexi	ST 36 zusanli	ST 40 fenlong	ST 42 chongyang
(SI) Small intestine	SI 1 shaoze	SI 2 qiangu	SI 3 houxi	SI 5 yanggu	SI 8 xiaohai	SI 7 zhizheng	SI 4 hand wangu
(BL) Bladder	BL 67 zhiyin	BL 66 tonggu	BL 65 shugu	BL 60 kunlun	BL 40 weizhong	BL 58 feiyang	BL 64 jinggu
(TE) Triple energizer	TE 1 guanchong	TE 2 yemen	TE 3 zhongzhu	TE 6 zhigou	TE 10 tianjing	TE 6 waiguan	TE 4 yangchi
(GB) Gall bladder	GB 44 foot qiaoyin	GB 43 xiaxi	GB 41 foot linqi	GB 38 yangfu	GB 34 yanglinguan	GB 37 guangming	GB 40 qiuxu

Table 3.3   Eight influential points

Zang Organs	(LR 13) *zhangmen*
Fu organs	(CV 12) *zhongwan*
Qi (Respiratory system)	(CV 17) *shanzhong*
Blood	(BL 17) *geshu*
Tendon	(GB 34) *yanglinguan*
Bone	(BL 11) *dashu*
Marrow	(GB 39) *xuanzhong*
Arterial pulse	(LU 9) *taiyuan*

3.5.1 Tonification point

This is the point which is used to draw *qi* from the 'Mother to Son' on the *Sheng* Cycle. It is the element point of the 'Mother' organ, e.g. the Metal point BL 67 (*zhiyin*) on the bladder meridian will draw *qi* from the LI into the BL.

3.5.2 Sedation point

This is the element point of the Son, e.g. if there is a need to reduce the *qi* in the BL, the Wood point (which is the 'Son') on the bladder meridian would be treated, i.e. the Wood point of the bladder is BL 65 (*shugu*).

3.5.3 Horary point

This is the point of the same element of the meridian on which it lies, e.g. the Water point on the bladder meridian is BL 66 (*tonggu*). This can be effective in stimulating energy if used at the time of day when *qi* is passing through the meridian. Referring to the 24-hour cycle (Figure 3.1), *qi* is at its greatest in the bladder between 15.00 and 17.00 hours. Thus, in clinical practice, if the patient attends for treatment at this time, BL 66 would be an effective point in stimulating bladder energy. Generally the horary point can be used at any time as an alternative to the source point.

3.5.4 Source/*yuang* point

This point is used to stimulate energy in a meridian without involving other meridians. In the *yin* (*zang*) organs this point is the Earth point, e.g. this would be KI 3 (*taixi*) in the kidney meridian. In the *fu* organs however, there is a separate source point, e.g. BL 64 (*jinggu*) in the bladder meridian.

3.5.5 *He-se* or *ho* point

Different schools of acupuncture use the term *he-se* or *ho* point. There is no difference in what the two words describe, but in this text the word *ho* will be used.

This is the most proximal command point, i.e. nearest the knee or elbow. Beyond this point the meridians pass deep into the tissues and are more difficult to 'tap'.

The *qi* in the meridian concentrates on this point and thus its major function is to facilitate the passage of *qi* through the meridian. It is used as a distal point when points along the meridian are being treated.

An example of the inclusion of a *ho* point in a treatment could be in a diagnosis of 'stuck' *qi* causing low back pain.

Local points on the bladder meridian would be pierced and then BL 40 (*weizhong*) which is the *ho* point would be treated, thus drawing the *qi* through the meridian and unblocking the channel.

It is one of the rules of acupuncture that when treating acupoints in the course of the meridian the *ho* point is also treated.

Some of the *ho* points have a wider significance for the whole body as well as their local meridian function, e.g. BL 40 (*weizhong*) is significant in skin conditions and GB 34 (*yanglinguan*) has an influence on muscles and ligaments as well as being the *ho* point of the gall bladder meridian.

3.5.6 *Tsing* point

This is the point that is sited at the lateral or medial side of the nail bed in the hands and feet. It is either the first or last point of the meridian. In the hand they are the first numbered points in the SI, LI, TE (*fu* organs) and in the foot the last numbered points BL, GB, ST (*fu* organs).

The opposite is the case with the *zang* organs, i.e. in the hand they are the last numbered points of the HT, PC, LU, and in the foot the first numbered points KI, SP, LR.

They can be used as an 'end' point when treating the point at the other end of the meridian, e.g. in treating a headache one could pierce GB 1 (*tongziliao*) and GB 44 (foot *qiaoyin*) drawing the *qi* from forehead to foot.

These *zing* or nail points are where the meridians are at their most superficial and when stimulated can achieve speedy results. Heating these points using moxabustion can quickly transmit heat energy into the full course of the meridian. In China, keeping the fingers and toes warm in cold weather conditions takes on a different significance than in the West. Vital *qi* can be lost through the nail points if allowed to get cold.

3.5.7 *Lo* point

This is the junction point of the paired organs and can be used to facilitate the passage of *qi* from one organ to the other using the transverse *lo* meridian. For example, if the kidney is weak and the bladder strong the *lo* (KI 4 *dazhong*) point of the kidney can be used to move the *qi* from the bladder to the kidney. If the reverse is the case, then the *lo* point of the bladder 58 (*feiyang*) can be treated.

The *lo* point can be used to move energy from the *yin* to *yang* paired organ prior to manipulating the *qi* using the *sheng* (Mother/Son) cycle. It also gives access to the long (longitudinal) *lo* meridians.

3.6 THE *LO* MERIDIANS

The description of the therapeutic use of the *lo* point in the previous section needs to be further examined. There are two meridian systems associated with these points. They are:

1. The tranverse *lo* meridians.
2. The long *lo* meridians.

Knowledge of the symptomatology of these systems is important to the clinician in order to make a proper diagnosis. If correctly used the *lo* point can be very useful; but one must be quite sure of the diagnosis, to ensure that one is manipulating the internal balance of *qi* and not moving **perverse** *qi*, (which has the effect of increasing the perceived fullness of the pulse), from one organ to another.

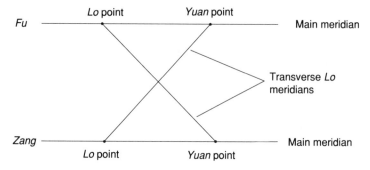

Figure 3.2 Diagram of transverse *lo* meridians.

3.6.1 Transverse *lo* meridians

These are the meridians which connect the *yuan* (source) point of one organ to the *lo* point of the paired organ (Figure 3.2). The differentiation of symptoms is summarized below.

LU: Perverse energy invasion:
   dyspnoea
   fullness of lungs
   pains in apex of lungs
   Internal causes:
   fullness in chest
   sensation of energy rising
   cough
   asthma
   hot palms of hands

LI: Perverse energy invasion:
   swelling of the neck
   ache in teeth
   Internal causes:
   dryness of mouth and throat
   pain along pathway LI 6 (*pianli*)–LU 9 (*taiyuan*)
   shivering (when very deficient)

ST: Perverse energy invasion:
   photophobia
   emotional feelings of wanting to be left alone
   borborygmus (rumbling tummy!)

Internal causes:
fever with sweating
catarrh
oedema of throat
abdominal distension
pain along pathway ST 40 (*fenglong*)–SP 3 (*taibai*)
fullness: heat in stomach and chest
dark urine
empty: cold in stomach and chest
and swollen stomach

SP: Perverse energy invasion:
abdominal distension with flatus
vomiting after meals
stiffness at root of tongue
Internal causes:
diarrhoea
pain in cardiac area
generalized feeling of stiffness
pain at root of tongue
disturbance on pathway SP 4 (*gongsun*)–ST 42 (*chongyang*)

HT: Perverse energy invasion:
dry throat with thirst
pain in cardiac area worse 23.00–1.00 hours
(NB this is when *qi* should be at its minimum in the HT
being 12 h after *qi* is passing through the HT)
Internal causes:
pains on pathway HT 5 (*tongli*)–SI 4 (hand *wangu*)

SI: Perverse energy invasion:
acute pains on pathway SI 7 (*zhizheng*)–HT 7 (*shenmen*)
Internal causes:
pain on whole pathway
tinnitus and/or deafness
submaxillary swelling

BL: Perverse energy invasion:
pains on pathway BL 58 (*feiyang*)–KI 3 (*taixi*)
Internal causes:
sharp pain along pathway
sharp pains in head and neck
yellowish eyes
lacrimation
haemorrhoids

KI: Perverse energy invasion:
cough; dyspnoea
hunger without being able to eat
visual disturbances
fearful and anxious
Internal causes:
pains along pathway KI 4 (*Dazhong*)–BL 64 (*jinggu*)
cold and numbness of legs
feeling of rising energy
dryness of throat and tongue
diarrhoea
grief

PC: Perverse energy invasion:
Hot palms combined with pain on pathway PC 6 (*neiguan*)–
TE 4 (*yangchi*)
forced laughter
red complexion
Internal causes:
circulatory disturbance
pain in heart
hot palms

TE: Perverse energy invasion:
sore throat
tinnitus and/or deafness
Internal causes:
pains on pathway TE 5 (*waiguan*)–PC 7 (*daling*)
perspiration

GB: Perverse energy invasion:
bitter taste in mouth
heat along line of meridian
Internal causes:
pains along pathway GB 37 (*guangming*)–LR 3 (*taichong*) and
in joints
sweating and shivering

LR: Perverse energy invasion:
pain in kidney area and stiffness of spine
genital infections
dry throat
Internal causes:
indigestion with nausea and vomiting
fullness in chest

diarrhoea
either urgency or retention of urine

3.6.2 The long *lo* meridians

A brief description of these meridians is given, together with a list of possible symptoms which may manifest themselves, when there is a disturbance in the long *lo* meridians. The *lo* point is identified for each organ.

Lung: LU 7 (*lieque*)
Passes into palm of hand and thenar eminence to connect with LI.
Excess: Hot palms.
Deficiency: Yawning and urinary frequency.

Large intestine: LI 6 (*pianli*)
Passes from LI and along the arm to LI 15 (*jianyu*), and ascends to the neck to the lower jaw, where it divides into two branches, one travelling to the roots of the teeth, the other to the ear.
Excess: Dental caries, deafness.
Deficiency: Cold sensation in teeth, feeling of oppression and pain in chest.

Stomach: ST 40 (*fenglong*)
Passes up from ST 40 along the lateral edge of the tibia through the abdomen and chest to GV 20 (*baihui*) and then decsends to the throat.
Excess: Dementia.
Deficiency: Weakness of joints in lower limbs and stiffness of the feet.
When this meridian is disordered it causes an inverse flow of energy which could lead to laryngeal blockage and sudden loss of voice.

Spleen: SP 4 (*gongsun*)
Passes from SP 4 up into the abdomen where it connects with the intestines and stomach.
Excess: Shooting pain in the abdomen.
Deficiency: Distension of abdomen.
When this meridian is disordered it causes an inverse flow of energy to the stomach and intestines causing diarrhoea.

Heart: HT 5 (*tongli*)
Runs parallel to main meridian to heart, tongue and eyes.

Excess *qi*: Produces a feeling of fullness around the diaphragm
   area.
Deficiency: Inability to speak.

Small intestine: SI 7 (*zhizheng*)
Runs up to the shoulders and heart.
Excess: Pain in shoulder and elbow joint.
Deficiency: Pimples.

Bladder: BL 58 (*feiyang*)
Runs into the main meridian from BL 58.
Excess: Blocked nose, pain along meridian line.
Deficiency: Epistaxis.

Kidney: KI 4 (*dazhong*)
Runs into the bladder meridian from KI 4. When it reaches the
abdomen it goes deep and radiates to the lumbar area and spine.
Excess: Retention of natural discharges, e.g. urine and stools.
Deficiency: Pain in lumbar region.
NB Any disturbance could give rise to chest problems.

Pericardium: PC 6 (*neiguan*)
Follows the main meridian pathway up the arm, penetrating deep
to the heart area.
Excess: Heart pain.
Deficiency: Stiff neck.

Triple energizer: TE 5 (*waiguan*)
Ascends the arm to the shoulder and penetrates deep to the chest
where it unites with the TE and pericardium.
Excess: Stiffness of the elbow.
Deficiency: Hyper-mobile elbow joint.

Gall bladder: GB 37 (*guangming*)
Travels down from GB 37 to the dorsum of the foot.
Excess: Coldness in the legs below the knee.
Deficiency: Unable to rise from sitting to standing due to loss of
   muscle power in the feet.

Liver: LR 5 (*ligou*)
Excess: Expanded swollen scrotum and penis.
Deficiency: Irritation of the scrotum.

Conception vessel: CV 15 (*jiuwei*)
Spreads out over abdomen from CV 15.
Excess: Painful skin.
Deficiency: Gnawing sensation in abdomen.

Governor: GV 1 (*changqiang*)
Passes up vertebral column to head and neck, then to the shoulder, scapula and through the bladder meridian to the renal and genital area.
Excess: Rigid spinal column.
Deficiency: Heavy head.

The symptomatology described above for the transverse *lo* and longitudinal *lo* vessels illustrates the complex nature of diagnosis faced with certain presenting symptoms.

How to manipulate energy using the lo *points*

In clinical practice, knowledge of these other (collateral) channels of energy can greatly enhance the efficacy of treatment. If one needs to treat energy disorders in the long *lo* vessels the simple principle is:

Excess: Drain the *lo* point of the meridian.
Deficiency: This is more complicated.
The long *lo* meridian is now lacking *qi*. The main meridian has taken up the perverse energy from it and thus is in a state of fullness. The *yuan* point is therefore sedated, but this via the transverse *lo* meridian will sedate the *lo* point of the paired organ. Therefore the coupled *lo* point should be supplied.

3.6.3 The tendino-muscular meridians

These meridians form a superficial network over the whole body and carry *wei* energy. This is the protective energy that is the first line of defence against perverse external influences.

They are so called because their pathways lie between the tendons and muscles. They roughly conform to the path of the main meridian to which they are associated.

Their common connection point with the main meridian is the *tsing* or nail point. Thus, energy runs up the arms and legs in all cases, unlike the main meridians whose energy flows alternately up and down the limbs and trunk, as described earlier in this chapter. It is at the *tsing* point that perverse energy, e.g. Heat or Cold, can invade the system and it is the tendino-muscular (TM) meridian that repels the invasion initially. If,

however, the *wei* energy is depleted, the perverse energy penetrates first into the TM and then to the main meridian. It is only when the perverse *qi* has penetrated the main meridian that it can be detected in the pulses.

The *wei* energy behaves differently in these meridians compared to the main channels. It flows in the *yang* (*fu*) meridians during the day and in the *yin* (*zang*) meridians at night.

(a) Symptomology of the tendino-muscular meridians

The affinity of the tendino-muscular meridians to the muscles and joint governs the symptoms experienced when there is a disturbance of energy in these superficial channels.

Aching muscles and joints are the main symptoms that a patient will describe and these will depend on whether there is Full or Empty condition.

Full
If the skin feels warm and pain can be elicited with only a light pressure, this indicates a Full condition. It follows that this is balanced by an Empty condition in the main meridian to preserve balance.

Empty
In this case there would not be pain on superficial pressure but there would be pain on deep palpation of the area and joint movement would be painful. This indicates a penetration of perverse energy into the main meridian.

(b) Treatment of tendino-muscular (TM) disorders

Full
Superficial needling of *ah shi* (tender) points is indicated to sedate the TM meridian, accompanied by supplying of the main meridian, either by using the *yuan* (source) point or the tonification point.

Empty
In this situation the main meridian should be sedated and the TM meridian supplied. For example, pain in the elbow joint on movement. Heat could be applied to the surface of the

elbow, using a hot pack. This will have a supplying effect superficially. LI 4 (*hegu*) could then be needled using a sedating technique.

Comment

Knowledge of the symptoms experienced when there is a disorder of the TM meridians is very useful in clinical practice especially when treating musculo-skeletal problems. Noninvasive techniques can be combined with needling when endeavouring to balance the energy (*qi*) between the main and TM meridians.

3.6.4 The distinct or divergent meridians

These are yet another defensive system associated with the main channels carrying only *wei* energy. They start superficially and then travel deep into the body to take defensive *wei qi* to the organs via pathways roughly parallel with the main meridians.

When perverse energy penetrates to the main meridian it can be transported to the governing organ, if the *jung* energy in the main channel is not sufficient to withstand it. The *wei* energy can help to divert some of the perverse energy into the distinct meridian and reduce the damage to the organ. The resulting symptoms will be less severe.

The paired distinct meridians all meet at a point on the head or neck, i.e.

BL and KI at BL 10 *tianzhu*
GB and LR at GB 1 *tongziliao*
ST and SP at BL 1 *jingming*
SI and HT at BL 1 *jingming*
TE and PC at TE 16 *tianyou*
LI and LU at LI 18 Neck *futu*

All the *yang* meridians in their turn meet at GV 20 *bahui*, thus one could say that at this point the entire network of the meridian system meets. NB In clinical practice there are some practitioners who always include GV 20 *bahui* in a treatment formula because of its influence on the meridian system.

Wei *energy in the distinct/divergent meridians*

The distinct and TM meridians differ in that *wei* energy which is carried in the Distinct system has a different pattern of behaviour to normal circulating *qi*.

It is active in the *yang* meridians during the day and in the *yin* meridians at night. It circulates alternately through the *yang* and *yin* meridians, i.e. BL, KI, GB, LR, ST, SP, SI, HT, TE, PC, LI, LU and into the BL again.

Signs and symptoms
Symptoms experienced by a patient are the result of the body's protective action against the perverse energy rather than to the actual perverse energy itself. Thus the severity of the symptoms will vary as *wei* energy fluctuates in the superficial and deep energic layers of the body.

Treatment
When perverse energy invades the meridian on one side of the body, it can flow via GV 20 *bahui* to the opposite side. It is important when trying to rid the body of the perverse energy, that the already reduced *jung* energy in the main meridian is not further depleted. The way to deal with this problem is to needle the *tsing*/nail point on the opposite side to the affected Distinct meridian to stimulate *wei* energy in the TM meridian without draining the *jung* energy from the main channel. For example, if the left distinct bladder meridian is affected, fluctuating pain on the left side of the head and neck may be the presenting symptom. The treatment should include BL 67 *zhiyin* on the right foot.

Conclusions
The above meridians are sometimes known collectively as the 'collaterals' of the main meridians. They do not register on the pulses and a careful history needs to be taken in order to identify the level of penetration of the perverse energy before deciding on a treatment programme.

3.7 THE 12 MAIN MERIDIANS

In this section an outline will be given of the course of each meridian and some of the more significant acupoints and symptomology discussed.

The location of the acupoints are described by identifying anatomical landmarks and measuring the distance from these landmarks by using the *'cun'* measurement. This takes into account the individual's height and build (Figure 5.3). A guide as to how deep the acupoint can be found is given in centimetres. This measurement can only be approximate, as the actual depth will be dependent on the amount of fatty tissue beneath the skin.

An indication of the angle of needle insertion is also given. These are illustrated in Figure 5.3, i.e. perpendicular 90°, oblique 45°, horizontal 15°.

The meridians are described in the same order as that of the circulation of *qi* through the *zang/fu* system, commencing with the Metal element and finishing with the Wood element.

3.7.1 Metal element (lung and large intestine meridians)

Tissue: skin
Sense organ: nose
Sense: smell

(a) Zang *organ*

Lung (LU) hand *taiyin* (Figure 3.3)

Linked with large intestine (LI)
Alarm point (*mu*): LU 1 *zhongfu*
Back *shu* point: BL 13 *feishu* 1.5 *cun* lateral to the spinous process of T3.
Maximal energy time: 3.00–5.00 hrs.

Course
There are 11 points identified along the course of this meridian. It commences on the lateral aspect of the chest 2 *cun* lateral to the nipple line and descends the arm on its antero-lateral aspect, passing over the thenar eminence to end at the lateral corner of the thumb nail.

Clinical applications
Symptoms associated with the respiratory system, skin, mucous membrane and local to the course of the channel.

Together with the SP it forms *tai yin* which is one of the inner layers of energy forming the Six *Chiaos*.

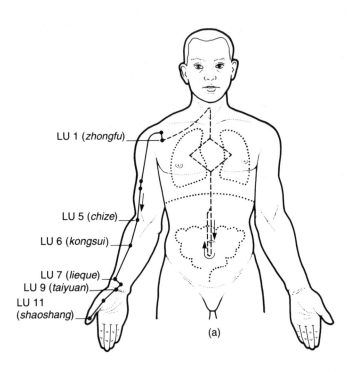

LU 1 (*zhongfu*)

LU 5 (*chize*)

LU 6 (*kongsui*)

LU 7 (*lieque*)
LU 9 (*taiyuan*)
LU 11
(*shaoshang*)

(a)

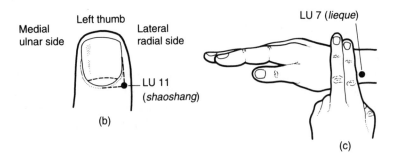

Medial
ulnar side

Left thumb

Lateral
radial side

LU 11
(*shaoshang*)

(b)

LU 7 (*lieque*)

(c)

Figure 3.3 The lung meridian (LU). The unbroken line indicates the main channel, the broken line shows internal connections.

Most significant points

- LU 1 *Zhongfu*
  Location: 2 *cun* lateral to the nipple line in the second inter-costal space.
  Indications:
  General: it eliminates Heat and regulates *qi*.
  Particular: this point is the alarm point of the lung. It is also useful for local shoulder problems. It should be nee-dled with great care as the lung lies immediately beneath this point.
  Puncture: 1.0–1.5 cm towards lateral aspect of chest.
- LU 5 *Chize, Ho* (*he-se*), sedative point. Location: on the lateral aspect of the anterior elbow crease lateral to the biceps tendon.
  Indications:
  General: eliminates pulmonary heat.
  Particular: this is a point to use in local problems or for sore throat and respiratory disorders. It can also be used as a remote point when other points on the lung channel are being treated.
  Puncture: perpendicularly 1.0–2.5 cm.
- LU 6 *Kongzui*: *Xi* cleft point.
  Location: on the radial aspect of the forearm 7 *cun* above wrist crease.
  Indications:
  General: eliminates pathogenic heat.
  Particular: this is useful for asthma, cough and tonsillitis. It is the *xi* cleft point and it can be used in acute problems in the lung.
  Puncture: perpendicularly 1.5–2.5 cm.
- LU 7 *Lieque, Lo* point connected to LI 4 (*hegu*) (Figure 3.3c).
  Location: on the radial side of the forearm, 1.5 *cun* proximal to the transverse wrist crease.
  Indications:
  General: removes pathogenic Wind and disperses pulmonary *qi*.
  Particular: this is a significant point for all lung conditions. It is the key point for *ren mai* which governs *yin* energy. Through its connection with LI 4 *hegu* via the *lo* meridian it can be of influence in LI meridian disturbances, e.g. tooth-ache, facial pain and paralysis.

Puncture: obliquely upwards 1.0–2.0 cm.
- LU 9 *Taiyuan* source point
  Location: in the depression on the radial side of the radial artery on the anterior wrist crease.
  Indications:
  General: influential point for the vascular system, e.g. arteriosclerosis and intermittent claudication.
  Particular: This is used for stimulating energy in the LU and as a local point, e.g. OA carpo-metacarpal joint.
  Puncture: perpendicularly 0.5–1.0 cm.
  Caution: point lies near to the radial artery!
- LU 11 *Shaoshang* tsing point
  Location: on the radial side of the thumb lateral to corner of nail (Figure 3.3b).
  Indications:
  General: eliminates pulmonary heat and is used in emergency to restore *yang qi*.
  Puncture: 0.2 cm.

(b) Fu *organ*

Large intestine (LI) hand *yangming* (Figure 3.4).

Linked with lung (LU)
Alarm point (*mu*): ST 25 (*tianshu*) 2 *cun* lateral to the umbilicus.
Back *shu* point: BL 25 (*dachlangshu*) 1.5 *cun* lateral to spinous process of L4/5.
Maximal energy time: 5.00–7.00 hrs.

Course
There are 20 acupoints on this meridian. It is a *yang* meridian and ascends from the lateral nail point of the index finger passing between the first and second metacarpals into the posterolateral aspect of the forearm and arm, crosses the shoulder joint from posterior to anterior and ascends the lateral side of the neck and crosses to the opposite side to terminate just lateral to the nasal ala.

Clinical applications: Symptoms associated with the colon and lung as well as the associated tissues, skin and mucous membrane.

Together with the ST it forms *yang ming* which is the deepest of the three outer layers of energy forming the Six *Chiaos*.

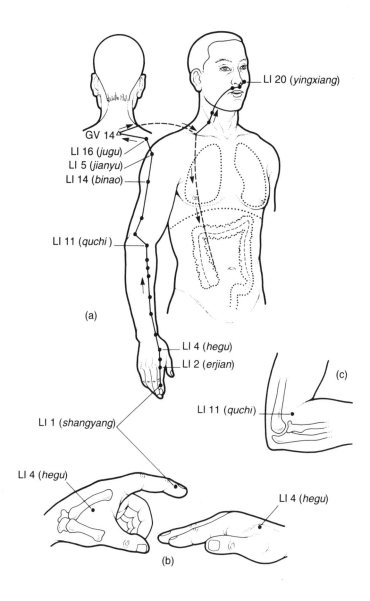

Figure 3.4 The large intestine meridian (LI). The unbroken line indicates the main channel, the broken line shows internal connections.

Most significant points

- LI 1 *shangyang* **tsing** point (Figure 3.4a,b)
  Location: sited opposite LU 11 medial to base of nail (Figure 3.3b).
  Indications:
  General: emergency point for reviving unconscious patient.
  Dispels heat.
  Particular: febrile diseases, parotitis, toothache.
  Puncture: 0.2 cm.

- LI 4 *hegu* source point connected via *lo* meridian to LU 7 (*lieque*) (Figures 3.3c and 3.4b)
  Location:
  (i) On the midpoint of a line connecting the 1st and 2nd metacarpal bones when the thumb is fully extended.
  (ii) Alternatively it is found on the highest point on the bulk of adductor pollicis when the thumb is adducted.
  Indications:
  General: it dispels Wind.
  Particular: it is a master point for pain in the body and is also used in anaesthesia.
  It has particular effect in low back pain and facial problems. Used with LR 3 (*taichong*) it has a calming and regulating effect on the whole body through stimulating the movement of blood and *qi*.
  Puncture: (i) perpendicularly 1–2 cm (ii) perpendicularly towards PC 8 *laogong*.

- LI 11 *quchi ho* point and tonification point (Figure 3.4c)
  Located: at lateral edge of elbow crease when elbow is flexed.
  Indications:
  General: reduces heat in ST and LI. It cools internal heat and eliminates Wind heat.
  This is a very useful point and is included in many treatments.
  Particular: it is an effective local point for the elbow. It is an immune enhancing point and is therefore incorporated in the treatment of such problems as hay fever and other allergies.
  It is used when patients are hypertensive/hypotensive and in endocrine disorders. It is also used as a remote point when other points are being treated on the large intestine channel.
  Puncture: perpendicularly towards HT 3 *shaohai* 2–3 cm.

- LI 14 *binao*
  Located: at the insertion of the deltoid into the humerus.
  Indications: used with other local points in shoulder pain.
  Puncture: perpendicularly 1–2 cm.
- LI 15 *jianyu*
  Location: at the antero-inferior border of the acromio-clavicular joint, inferior to the acromion process when arm is in adduction.
  Indications:
  General: eliminates penetrating Wind.
  Particular: this is often used in shoulder problems as a local point.
  Puncture: perpendicularly 1–2.5 cm when arm is in abduction or obliquely downwards 2–3 cm when arm is adducted.
- LI 16 *jugu*
  Location: in the depression between acromium and spine of scapula (Figure 3.4a).
  Indications: pain in shoulder, back and upper extremities.
  Puncture: 2–2.5 cm on a lateral oblique line.
- LI 20 *yingxiang*
  Location: between the naso-labial groove and the midpoint of the outer border of the nasal ala.
  Indications:
  General: dispels Wind heat.
  Particular: rhinitis, blocked nose, facial paralysis and toothache. It is used in conjunction with LI 4 *hegu* and LI 11 *quchi* in allergic conditions, e.g. hay fever.
  Puncture: obliquely towards nose 1–1.5 cm.

3.7.2 Earth element (stomach and spleen meridians)

Tissue: connective tissue
Sense organ: mouth
Sense: taste

(a) Fu *organ*

Stomach (ST) foot *yangming* (Figure 3.5).

Linked with spleen (SP)
Alarm point *mu*: CV 12 (*zhongwan*)

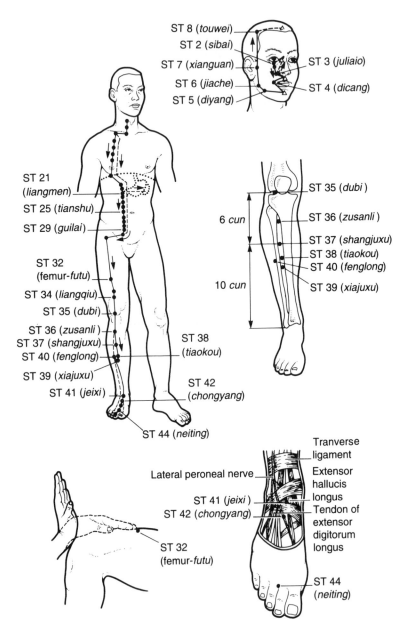

Figure 3.5 The stomach meridian (ST). The unbroken line indicates the main channel, the broken line shows internal connections.

Back *shu* point: BL21 (*weishu*) 1.5 *cun* lateral to T12.
Maximum energy time: 7.00–9.00 hrs.

Course of channel
There are 45 points identified along the stomach channel. The
first point is sited below the eyeball. The channel then descends
to the mandible, loops up to the hairline passing over the
tempero-mandibular joint, re-emerging half way down the
antero-lateral aspect of the neck. It then descends following a line
through the nipple 4 *cun* lateral to the midline of the sternum.
It next descends to the abdomen to 2 *cun* lateral to the midline
and thence to the groin. It re-emerges on the anterior aspect of
the upper thigh descending to the lateral nail point of the second
toe.

This meridian is unique in that it is the only *yang* meridian to be
situated on the anterior of the torso and abdomen.

Clinical applications
It has many clinical applications. These are concerned with the
areas local to the acupoints as well as significant effects on the
whole energic balance of the body, i.e. the points on the face are
used for facial pain, eye disorders and toothache. The points
in the thoracic area are rarely used, but can be considered for
chest pain and disorders of the mammary glands. The points on
the abdomen are used in abdominal and pelvic disorders. Those
in the leg can be used in the treatment for paralysis and joint
disorders.

Together with the LI it forms *yang ming* which is the deepest of
the three outer defensive layers of the Six *Chiaos*.

Most significant points
• ST 2 *sibai*
 Location: directly below ST 1 on the infra-orbital foramen.
 Indications:
 General: it dispels external and internal Wind.
 Particular: facial paralysis, eye disorders and trigeminal
  neuralgia.
 Puncture: perpendicularly 0.5–1.0 cm.
• ST 3 *juliao*
 Location: directly below ST 2 at the lower border of the ala
  nasi.

Indications: trigeminal neuralgia, sinusitis, rhinitis, toothache and facial paralysis.

This point is very tender when there is any congestion in the sinuses. Acupressure can give immediate relief.

Puncture: obliquely 0.5–1.0 cm.

- ST 4 *dicang*

Location: 0.4 *cun* lateral to the corner of the mouth.

Indications: local for paralysis of obicularis oris. Lower branch of trigeminal nerve in trigeminal neuralgia. Aphasia and hypersalivation.

Puncture: obliquely 1.0 cm or horizontally towards ST 6 *jiache* 2–4 cm.

- ST 5 *daying*

Location: at the lowest border of the masseter muscle.

Indications: trigeminal neuralgia, toothache, parotitis, facial paralysis.

Puncture: perpendicularly 0.5 cm.

- ST 6 *jiache*

Location: at midpoint of masseter muscle when the jaw is closed.

Indications:

General: calms external and internal Wind and helps to remove heat in the *yang ming*.

Particular: trigeminal neuralgia, toothache, parotitis, trismus and facial paralysis.

Puncture: perpendicularly 0.5 cm.

- ST 7 *xianguan*

Location: in the depression on the lower border of the zygomatic arch, anterior to the condyloid process of the mandible. Should be located with the patient's mouth closed.

Indications: temporo-mandibular joint problems.

Puncture: perpendicularly 0.5–1.0 cm.

- ST 8 *touwei*

Location: 0.5 *cun* dorsal to the corner of the hairline directly above ST 7 *xianguan*.

Indications:

General: dispels Wind.

Particular: vertigo, migraine, frontal and parietal headache, excessive lacrimation.

It is an excellent emergency point for acupressure in cases of migraine/headaches.

Puncture: horizontally anterior or posterior depending on location of pain, 1 cm.

- ST 21 *liangmen*
  Location: 2 *cun* lateral to the midline, 4 *cun* above the umbilicus and lateral to CV 12 *zhongwan* with which it is often used.
  Indications:
  General: stimulates the stomach and spleen.
  Particular: it is used in acute and chronic gastritis, stomach and duodenal ulcers, gall bladder disorders, vomiting and nausea.
  Puncture: perpendicularly 1–2 cm. This point should be punctured with care.
- ST 25 *tianshu mu*/alarm point of large intestine
  Location: 2 *cun* lateral to the umbilicus.
  Indications:
  General: it stimulates the function of blood and *qi*. Diagnosis of large intestine disorders.
  Particular: acute and chronic gastric problems and nausea.
  Puncture: perpendicularly 1–2 cm.
  It is a good point to heat with ST 21 *liangmen* and CV 12 *zhongwan* using Moxa if the patient is debilitated.
- ST 29 *guilai*
  Location: 4 *cun* below ST 25 (*tianshu*) and 2 *cun* lateral to the midline.
  Indications:
  General: It moves stagnation of blood and *qi*.
  Particular: this point can be included with other abdominal points for urogenital disorders, constipation, diarrhoea, pelvic inflammation and dysmenorrhoea.
  Puncture: perpendicularly 1–2 cm.
- ST 32 femur *futu*
  Location: 6 *cun* above the superior border of the patella. If the patient's knee is flexed and the practitioner's wrist is placed over the mid point of the patella, the area under the tip of the middle finger is where the point is located.
  Indications: pain and paralysis of the leg.
  Puncture: 2–3 cm along lateral border of femur.
- ST 33 *yinshi*
  Location: in a depression above the supero-lateral border of the patella.
  Indications: pain in the knee, weakness in the leg.

Puncture: perpendicularly 2–3 cm.
- ST 34 *liangqiu*: *xi* cleft point
  Location: 1 *cun* below ST 33 *yinshi*.
  Indications:
  It stimulates movement of *qi* in the legs.
  This is the *xi* cleft point and is indicated for acute gastric and intestinal disorders. Also effective for gastralgia, diarrhoea, mastitis and problems of the knee joint.
  Puncture: perpendicularly 2 cm.
- ST 35 *dubi*
  Location: in a depression lateral to the lower border of the patella when the knee is slightly flexed.
  Indications:
  General: it removes blockages in the meridian.
  Particular: used for local knee disorders with extra point 32 *xiyan* which lies on the medial aspect of the lower border of the patella and extra point 31 *heding* on the superficial border of the patella.
  Puncture: obliquely medially 1–2 cm.
- ST 36 *zusanli ho* point
  Location: one finger breadth lateral to the tibial tubercle and 3 *cun* below ST 35 *dubi*.
  Indications:
  General: it regulates the circulation of blood and *qi*.
  Particular: it is an important distal point for abdominal disorders including gastritis, nausea, stomach and duodenal ulcers, constipation, diarrhoea and as a remote point when other points are being treated along the stomach channel.
  General tonification and homeostatic effects in metabolic disease. Relief of pain generally.
  It is one of the most used points in acupuncture with a wide range of effects.
  Puncture: perpendicularly 2–3 cm.
- ST 37 *shangjuxu*
  Location: 6 *cun* below ST 35 *dubi* and one finger width lateral to the anterior crest of the tibia.
  Indications:
  General: it can be used to balance energy when there is too much in the upper part of the body.
  Particular: it is the lower *ho* point of the LI. It can be used for

abdominal pain, diarrhoea and appendicitis as well as paralysis of the legs.

Puncture: perpendicularly 2–3 cm.

* ST 38 *tiaokou*
Location: 2 *cun* on a vertical line below ST 37 *shangjuxu*.
Indications:
This point is very useful in shoulder problems.
Puncture: perpendicularly 2–3 cm to obtain strong *deqi* then immediately move the shoulder.
* ST 39 *xiajuxu*
Location: 3 *cun* below ST 37 *shangjuxu*.
Indications:
Used when there is too little energy in the lower part of the body.
Puncture: perpendicularly 2 cm.
* ST 40 *fenglong lo* point connecting to SP 3 *Taibai*
Location: one finger width lateral to ST 38 *tiaokou* and 8 *cun* below ST 35.
Indications: Excessive white phlegm in bronchitis and bonchial asthma.
Puncture: perpendicularly 2–3 cm.
* ST 41 *jiexi* tonification point (Fire)
Location: on the midpoint of the dorsum of the foot at the transverse malleolus crease, between the tendons of extensor digitorum and extensor hallucis longus.
Indications: weakness of dorsi-flexion of the ankle and local point for ankle.
Puncture: perpendicularly 0.5–1.0 cm.
* ST 42 *Chongyang*, source point connecting with SP 4 *gongsun* (via long. *lo* meridian)
Location: 1.5 *cun* distal to ST 41 *jiexi* on dorsum of foot where the artery can be palpated.
Indications: local problems in foot and can be used to relieve toothache.
Puncture: perpendicularly 0.5–1.0 cm avoiding the artery.
* ST 44 *neiting*, Water point
Location: 0.5 *cun* proximal to the web between the 2nd and 3rd metatarsals.
Indications: important point for toothache, headache, gastralgia, diarrhoea and general analgesia.
Puncture: perpendicular 0.5–1.0 cm.

(b) Zang *organ*

Spleen (SP), foot – *taiyin* (Figure 3.6).

Linked with **stomach** (ST).
Alarm point (*mu*): LR 13 *zhangmen* (tip of 11th rib).
Back *shu* point: BL 20 *pishu* 1.5 *cun* lateral to spinous process of
    T 11.
Maximum energy time: 9.00–11.00 hrs.

Course
There are 21 points along the course of this meridian. It starts at
the medial nail point of the hallux, passes along the medial border
of the foot and ascends the medial aspect of the leg to the medial
area below the knee joint. It then ascends the thigh and emerges in
the abdomen 4 *cun* lateral to the midline. It then passes up to the
second intercostal space and descends to finish in the 6th intercostal space on the axillary line.

Clinical applications
The functions of the spleen include the pancreas and its secretions. It has application to the function of the spleen and the
reticuloendothelial system. Traditionally the spleen also regulates
the water and blood metabolism to influence the connective tissue, lips and tongue.
    The spleen points are used in treating digestive, urogenital and
skin disorders.
    Together with the LU it forms the *tai yin*. It is one of the deeper
layers of energy forming one of the Six *Chiaos*.

Most Significant Points

- SP 2 *dadu* tonification point (Fire)
    Location: on the medial side of the great toe, anterior and
        inferior to the 1st metacarpo-phalangeal (MTP) joint.
    Indications:
    General: abdominal pain/distension.
    Particular: used with SP 3 *taibai* in local treatment for arthritis
        of the 1st MTP joint.
    Puncture: perpendicularly 0.5–1.0 cm.
- SP 3 *taibai* source point (earth) connecting with ST 40 *fenglong*
    (transverse *lo* meridian).

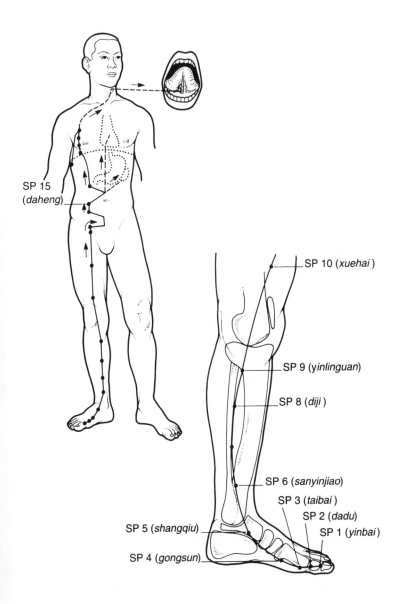

Figure 3.6 The spleen meridian (SP). The unbroken line indicates the main channel, the broken line shows internal connections.

Location: posterior and inferior to the head of the 1st metacarpal.

Indications:

General: gastralgia, diarrhoea, vomiting and constipation.

Particular: used with SP 2 *dadu* for local treatment of 1st MTP joint.

Puncture: perpendicularly 0.5–1.0 cm.

- SP 4 *gongsun lo* point, connecting with ST 42 *chongyang*.

Location: medial border of foot in a depression immediately distal to the base of the 1st metatarsal.

Indications:

General: its connection with the ST meridian means that it can influence areas that the ST meridian affects. It is also the key point of *Chong Mai* which is one of the eight extra meridians and is therefore influential in urogenital problems.

Particular: acupressure/acupuncture can be effective in relieving low abdominal pain.

Puncture: perpendicularly 1–2 cm.

- SP 5 *shangqiu* sedation point (Metal)

Location: in hollow anterior and inferior to medial malleolus.

Indications:

General: abdominal distension.

Particular: local point for ankle problems.

Puncture: perpendicularly 0.5–1.0 cm.

- SP 6 *sanyinjiao*

Location: 3 *cun* above the medial malleolus and just posterior to the tibial border.

Indications:

General: invigorates the collateral meridians, regulates *qi* and blood.

Particular: this is a highly influential point. The three *yin* (KI SP LR) meridians of the leg meet in this area and are therefore influenced by this point. It traditionally balances the *yin* and *yang* energy of the kidney. It supports the abdominal viscera and is thus a master point for urogenital disorders including enuresis, nocturia and menstrual problems.

It is a general tonification point for the body and it can be stimulated to speed uterine contractions during labour and relieve pain.

It is a valuable point for insomnia.

Treatment note: this is a large point and can be easily palpated. It is important to feel if the area is soft or tense. This local palpation will decide on the method of stimulation. If soft the treatment needs to be a supplying one, if tense then a 'reducing' technique is required. NB The supplying technique could be heating with Moxa.

Puncture: perpendicular 1–2.5 cm.

- SP 8 *diji xi* cleft point
  Location: 3 *cun* below SP 9 *yinlingquan* at the posterior border of the tibia.
  Indications: this is the *xi* cleft point and is effective in acute spleen problems. Also indicated for lumbago, mennorrhagia and abdominal distension.
  Puncture: perpendicularly 2–4 cm.

- SP 9 *yinlingquan ho* point
  Location: in a depression just below the medial condyle of the tibia on a level with the tuberosity of the tibia.
  Indications:
  General: eliminates heat, resolves damp.
  Particular: local to the knee, irregular menstruation and abdominal distension and enuresis.
  As a remote point when other points on the spleen meridian are being treated.
  Puncture: perpendicularly 2–3 cm or directed posteriorly toward GB 34 *yanglinguan*.

- SP 10 *xuehai*
  Location: 2 *cun* proximal to the upper border of patella at the highest point of the vastus medialis muscle.
  Indications:
  General: eliminates Wind, dispels heat and regulates the circulation of *qi* and blood.
  Particular: traditionally this is the point for cooling the blood. It is used in skin conditions which are hot and irritating, also urogenital disorders.
  Puncture: perpendicularly 2–3 cm.

- SP 15 *daheng*
  Location: 4 *cun* lateral to umbilicus and level with ST 25 *tianshu*.
  Indications: abdominal pain, gastritis, dyspepsia and constipation.
  Puncture: perpendicularly 1–2 cm.

3.7.3 Fire element (heart and small intestine meridians)

Tissue: blood and blood vessels
Sense organ: tongue
Sense: speech

(a) Zang *organ*

Heart (HT), hand *shaoyin* (Figure 3.7).

Alarm point (*mu*): CV 14 *jujue*
Back *shu* point: BL 15 *xinshu*. 1.5 *cun* lateral to spinous process of T5.
Maximum energy time: 11.00–13.00 hrs.

Course
There are nine points identified along the heart channel.

The first point is sited in the axilla and the meridian descends the antero-medial arm and forearm, crosses the palm and ends at the nail point on the radial side of the little finger.

Clinical application
Traditionally the heart organ not only controls the circulation and function of the heart, but also the brain and consciousness. Thus the points identified on this meridian are used in psychological problems and are also effective for symptoms local to the meridian.

Together with the *ki* it forms the deepest of the Six *Chiaos, chao yin*.

In clinical practice this meridian is treated with great respect as the acupoints have a profound effect on heart function.

Most significant points
* HT 3 *shaohai*, source point
  Location: between the medial end of the transverse cubital crease and the medial epicondyle of the humerus when elbow is bent.
  Indications:
  General: dispels pathogenic heat from the heart, calms the mind and resolves phlegm.
  Particular: numbness of forearm and hand; angina pectoris and local elbow problems.

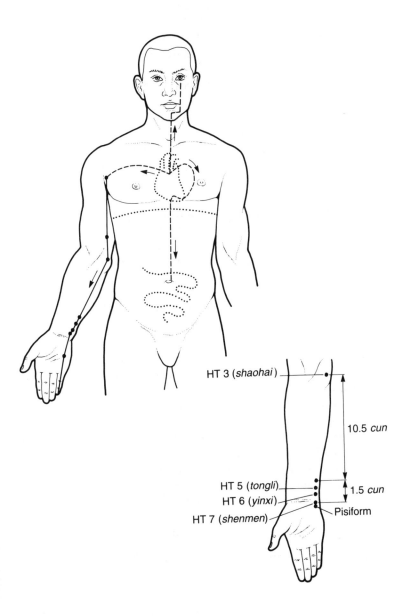

Figure 3.7 The heart meridian (HT). The unbroken line indicates the main channel, the broken line shows internal connections.

Puncture: perpendicularly 1–2 cm.

- HT 5 *tongli lo* point connecting to SI 4 hand *wangu*.

    Location: on the ulnar side of the wrist, on the radial side of the tendon of flexor carpi ulnaris, 1 *cun* proximal to HT 7 *shenmen*.

    Indications: speech disturbances, sudden hoarseness and insomnia.

    Puncture: perpendicularly 0.5–1.0 cm.

- HT 6 *yinxi, xi* cleft point.

    Location: 0.5 *cun* proximal to HT 7 *shenmen*.

    Indications: angina pectoris, night sweating and acute cardiac disorders.

    Puncture: 0.5–1.0 cm.

- HT 7 *shenmen*, sedative point and source point connecting to SI 7 *zhizheng* via tranverse *lo* meridian.

    Location: on the transverse crease of the wrist in the depression at the radial side of the tendon of flexor carpi ulnaris, just posterior to the pisiform.

    Indications:

    General: removes obstruction from the meridian and calms the mind and heart.

    Particular: hysteria, insomnia, poor memory.

    This is a very useful point to use in any situation which involves stress and anxiety. It is a point that a patient can be shown how to stimulate with acupressure, in times of stress or insomnia due to the mind racing.

- HT 9 *shaochong*, tonification point.

    Location: on the radial side of the little finger 0.1 *cun* proximal to the base of the nail.

    Indications: acute situations involving the heart and circulation, acute chest pain and coma.

    Puncture: perpendicularly 0.3 cm.

(b) Fu *organ*

Small intestine SI hand – *Taiyang* (Figure 3.8).

Linked with Heart (HT).

Alarm point (*mu*): CV 4 *guanyuan*.

Back *shu* point: BL 27 *xiaochangshu* 1.5 *cun* lateral to spinous process of S1.

Maximum energy time: 13.00–15.00 hrs.

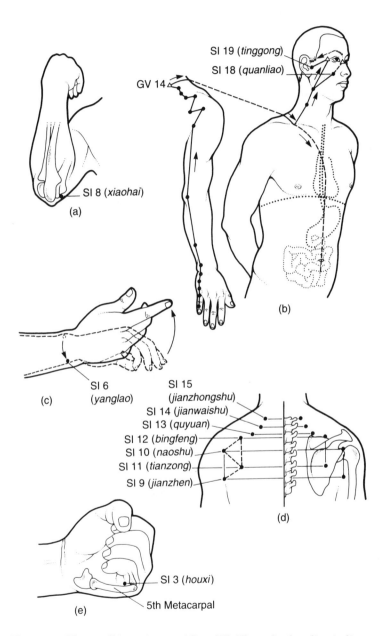

Figure 3.8 The small intestine meridian (SI). The unbroken line indicates the main channel, the broken line shows internal connections.

Course
The channel starts at the corner of the little finger nail on the ulnar side, passes upwards on the ulnar and dorsal aspect of the forearm and arm to the posterior aspect of the shoulder. It then traces a zigzag course into the lateral aspect of the cervical spine to the cheek and finishes anterior to the ear.

Clinical applications
Treatment of painful disorders local to the path of the meridian. These include periarthritis of the shoulder, toothache, trigeminal neuralgia and ear disorders.

The small intestine together with the bladder meridian form the *Tai Yang* axis, which is the most superficial of the Six *Chiaos*.

Most Significant Points
- ST 3 *houxi* tonification point, key point of *du mai*.
  Location: at the end of the transverse crease proximal to the 5th metacarpo-phalangeal joint when hand is half clenched.
Indications:
General: eliminates internal Wind-Heat.
Particular: stiffness or rigidity of neck, tinnitus, deafness, occipital headache and lumbago.
It is the key point of *du mai* and used with BL 62 *shenmai*, the key point of *yang chiao mai*. It is said to affect the autoimmune system and can be used in a treatment plan for rheumatoid arthritis.
  Puncture: perpendicularly 1–2 cm.
- SI 5 *yanggu horary* point.
  Location: at the ulnar side of the wrist in the depression between the ulnar styloid and the pisiform bone.
  Indications:
  General: regulates SI *qi*.
  Particular: pain in the lateral aspect of arm and wrist. It can also be used for tonifying the SI.
  Puncture: perpendicularly 0.5–1.0 cm.
- SI 6 *yanglao xi* cleft point.
  Location: in the depression on the radial side of the styloid process of the ulna (Figure 3.8c).
  Indications:

General: acute disorders of SI channel.

Puncture: obliquely 2–2.5 cm towards PC 6 (*neiguan*)

- SI 8 *xiaohai ho* point.

  Location: in the posterior aspect of the cubital joint, in a depression between the olecranon of the ulna and the tip of the medial epycondyle of the humerus (Figure 3.8a).

  Indications: pain in small finger, elbow and shoulder. It can also be used as a remote point on the SI channel.

  Puncture: perpendicularly 0.5–1.0 cm.

- SI 9 *jianzhen*

  Location: with arm at the side it is 1 *cun* above the dorsal crease of the axilla (Figure 3.8d).

  Indications: periarthritis of the shoulder, pain in the arm and paralysis of the arm.

  Puncture: perpendicularly 2–3 cm.

The following five points (SI 10–14) are all of value in treating pain in the scapula and upper fibres of trapezius (Figure 3.8d). They are often identified as trigger points and can be treated as such. In these cases the needling would be very superficial, as for the tendino-muscular meridians (see Chapter 10 on trigger point acupuncture).

- SI 10 *naoshu*

  Location: with arm at the side it is directly above the posterior axilla fold on the lower border of the spine of scapula.

  Puncture: obliquely towards lateral aspect 2–3 cm.

- SI 11 *tianzong*

  Location: in the centre of the infra-scapular fossa forming a triangle with SI 10 *naoshu* and SI 9 *jianzhen*.

  Indications:

  General: eliminates stagnant *qi* from chest.

  Puncture: perpendicularly 1–2 cm.

- SI 12 *bingfeng*

  In the centre of the supra-scapular fossa above SI 11 *tianzong*.

  Puncture: obliquely 1–2 cm.

- SI 13 *quyuan*

  Location: on the medial end of the supra-scapular fossa midway between SI 10 *naoshu* and the spinous process of the 2nd thoracic vertebra.

  Puncture: obliquely 1–2 cm.

- SI 14 *jianweishu*
  Location: 3 *cun* lateral to the lower border of the spinous
  process of the 1st thoracic vertebra.
  Puncture: obliquely 1–2 cm.
- SI 15 *jianzhongshu*
  Location: 2 *cun* lateral to the lower border of the 7th cervical
  vertebra.
  Indications: besides its local musculo-skeletal effect, it is a
  useful point in bronchitis and asthma.
  Puncture: obliquely 1–2 cm.
- SI 18 *quanliao*
  Location: directly below the outer canthus, in the depression
  below the lower border of the zygomatic arch (Figure 3.8b).
  Indications:
  General: dispels Wind.
  Particular: facial paralysis, toothache and trigeminal
  neuralgia.
  Puncture: perpendicularly 0.5–1.0 cm.
- SI 19 *tinggong*
  Location: in the depression shown between the tragus and
  TMJ when the mouth is slightly open.
  Indications:
  General: removes obstruction from meridian.
  Particular: tinnitus, deafness, earache.
  Puncture: 1–2 cm.

3.7.4 Water element (bladder and kidney meridians)

Season: winter
Tissue: bones and joints
Sense organ: ear
Sense: hearing

(a) Fu *organ*

Bladder (BL) foot *taiyang* (Figure 3.9).
Linked with the kidney (KI)
Alarm point (*mu*): CV 3 *zhongji*
Back *shu* point: BL 28 *pangguangshu* 1.5 *cun* lateral to the spinous
process of S2.
Maximum energy time: 15.00–17.00 hrs.

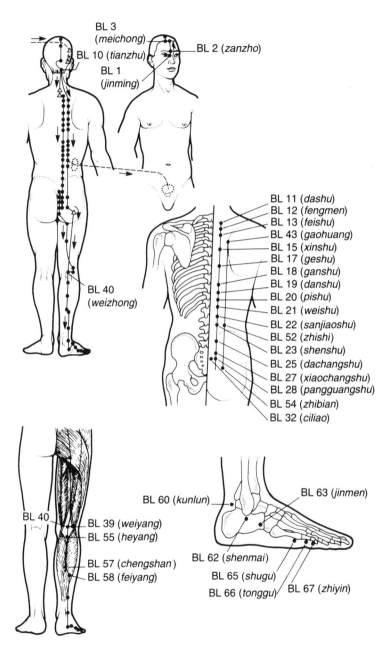

BL 3 (*meichong*)
BL 10 (*tianzhu*)
BL 1 (*jinming*)
BL 2 (*zanzho*)

BL 40 (*weizhong*)

BL 11 (*dashu*)
BL 12 (*fengmen*)
BL 13 (*feishu*)
BL 43 (*gaohuang*)
BL 15 (*xinshu*)
BL 17 (*geshu*)
BL 18 (*ganshu*)
BL 19 (*danshu*)
BL 20 (*pishu*)
BL 21 (*weishu*)
BL 22 (*sanjiaoshu*)
BL 52 (*zhishi*)
BL 23 (*shenshu*)
BL 25 (*dachangshu*)
BL 27 (*xiaochangshu*)
BL 28 (*pangguangshu*)
BL 54 (*zhibian*)
BL 32 (*ciliao*)

BL 40

BL 60 (*kunlun*)
BL 63 (*jinmen*)
BL 39 (*weiyang*)
BL 55 (*heyang*)
BL 57 (*chengshan*)
BL 58 (*feiyang*)
BL 62 (*shenmai*)
BL 65 (*shugu*)
BL 66 (*tonggu*)
BL 67 (*zhiyin*)

Figure 3.9 The bladder meridian (BL). The unbroken line indicates the main channel, the broken line shows internal connections.

Course

There are 67 acupoints identified along the course of this meridian. It starts at the inner canthus of the eye, ascends the forehead and passes over the frontal bone and down to occiput 0.5 *cun* from the midline. It then divides into two branches. The more medial branch descends from T1 to S4 1.5 *cun* lateral to the midline. The outer branch descends from T2 to S4 3 *cun* lateral to the midline. The inner branch ascends from S4 to the first sacral foramen and descends again to 0.5 *cun* lateral to the coccyx. It re-emerges at the midpoint of the gluteal fold and passes down the posterior aspect of the thigh to the midpoint of the knee crease where it joins again with the lateral branch. The combined meridian then descends between the medial and lateral bellies of the gastrocnemius, tracks lateral to the midline of the leg, passing inferior to the lateral malleolus along the lateral border of the foot, to terminate at the fifth toe 0.1 *cun* lateral to the nail.

Clinical applications

This meridian has many applications in clinical practice.

1. The outer branch which descends parallel to the inner branch is used traditionally, when there is a psychological reinforcement of the effect of using points on the medial branch. For example, if the point BL 23 *shenshu* is treated to affect the energy of the kidney, BL 52 *zhishi* will reinforce the effect if there is an element of fear in the symptoms presented. (Fear being the internal emotion of Water of which kidney is the *zang* organ).

2. Points throughout the length of this meridian can be used effectively in local problems.
   Those on the face, for eye disorders and headaches.
   Those on the occiput and neck, for occipital headache and cervical problems.

3. Some of those on the inner branch, which start at BL 13 *feishu* (level T3/4) and finish at BL 27 *xiaochangshu* (level L4/5) have a direct effect on specific parts of the body. These are the back *shu* points.

4. The points thoughout the length of the spine are also effective in local joint and soft tissue problems.

5. The points in the leg coincide to a large extent with the path of

the sciatic nerve. These are used in referred leg pain as well as in local joint and soft tissue problems.

The BL together with the TE form *tai yang*, the most superficial of the Six Chiaos.

Most significant points

- BL 1 *jingming*
  Location: 0.1 *cun* lateral and superior to the inner canthus near the medial orbital border.
  Indications:
  General: dispels internal Wind, eliminates heat.
  Particular: local eye problems.
  NB This is a difficult point to puncture and requires a highly skilled technique. For this reason many practitioners do not attempt to pierce this point. It is believed to stimulate the anterior pituitary and it is used in combination with SI 3 *houxi* (key point of *du mai*) and BL 62 *shenmai* (key point of *yang chiao mai*) to increase ACTH.
  Puncture: either 1–2 cm along orbital wall or superficially 0.3–0.5 cm.
- BL 2 *zanzhu*
  Location: directly above the inner canthus in a small hollow on the medial side of the brow.
  Indications:
  General: dispels Wind, calms the LR.
  Particular: eye disorders, frontal headache, migraine and frontal sinusitis. Some practitioners use this point instead of BL 1 claiming similar effects.
  Puncture: either 0.5–1.0 cm horizontally subcutaneously downward or laterally, or perpendicularly 0.5–1.0 cm.
- BL 3 *meichong*
  Location: directly above BL 2 *zanzhu* 0.5 *cun* inside the hairline.
  Indications: headache, blurring of vision and redness and swelling of eye.
  Puncture: obliquely 0.5–1.0 cm.
- BL 10 *tianzhu*
  Location: 1.3 *cun* lateral to the midline at level C1/2.

Indications:
General: dispels Wind, stimulates the meridians.
Particular: headache, cervical spondylosis and migraine.
This is an accessible point for patients to treat them-
selves using acupressure. It can sometimes abort an onset of
migraine or occipital headache if treated immediately.
Puncture: obliquely 0.5–1.0 cm.

NB The following acupoints described in the thoracic spine must
be needled with great care, to avoid piercing the pleura. This may
be a problem when treating cases of chronic lung disease such as
emphysema, when the pleura become more superficial due to
hypertrophy of the alveoli. Some practitioners needle these points
obliquely although the Chinese texts describe perpendicular
needle insertion.

• BL 11 *dashu*, influential point for bone.
  Location: 1.5 *cun* lateral to the lower border of the spinous
    process of T1.
  Indications:
  General: it is an influential point for bones. It can be used for
    osteoporosis and where there is delayed union following
    surgery or fracture.
  Particular: it is effective in acute bronchitis when combined
    with BL 12 *fengmen* and BL 13 *feishu*.
    It can be used for local pain.
  Puncture: perpendicularly 0.5–1.0 cm.
• BL 12 *fengmen*
  Location: 1.5 *cun* lateral to the lower border of the spinous
    process of T2.
  Indications:
  General: expels Wind. Helps circulation of *qi* and strengthens
    the dispersal function of the LU.
  Particular: local pain.
  Puncture: 0.5–1.0 cm.
• BL 13 *feishu, shu* point of the lung.
  Location: 1.5 *cun* lateral to the lower border of the spinous
    process of T3.
  Indications:
  General: dispels heat from the LU.
  Particular: chronic bronchitis, bronchial asthma.

This is a point which can be very effective when heated with Moxa if *yang* energy is low in the lung.
Puncture: perpendicularly 0.5–1.0 cm.

- BL 14 *jueyinshu shu* point of the pericardium.
  Location: 1.5 *cun* lateral to the lower border of the spinous process of T4.
  Indications: pain in the thorax and reinforcing *qi* in the PC.
  Puncture: perpendicularly 0.5–1.0 cm.
- BL 15 *xinshu shu* point of the heart.
  Location: 1.5 *cun* lateral to the lower border of the spinous process of T5.
  Indications:
  General: stimulates circulation of *qi* and blood.
  Particular: angina pectoris, mental disorders.
  Puncture: perpendicularly (with care) 0.5–1.0 cm.
- BL 16 *dushu shu* point of the Governor Vessel.
  Location: 1.5 *cun* lateral to the lower border of the spinous process of T6.
  Indications: any situation which requires a reinforcement of *qi* in the Governor Vessel.
  Puncture: this is a forbidden point to needle because of the nearness of the pleura to the skin surface. It can be treated with moxa.
- BL 17 *geshu shu* point of the diaphragm and influential for blood.
  Location: 1.5 *cun* lateral to the lower border of the spinous process of T7.
  Indications:
  General: stimulates circulation of blood. Strengthens the body as a whole and disperses fullness in the diaphragm.
  Particular: hiccough, nausea, bronchial asthma, disorders of the blood.
  Puncture: perpendicularly (with care) 0.5–1.0 cm.
- BL 18 *ganshu shu* point of the liver.
  Location: 1.5 *cun* lateral to the lower border of the spinous process of T9.
  Indications:
  General: eliminates damp-heat and stagnation of *qi*.
  Particular: liver and gall bladder disorders, eye problems.
  Puncture: perpendicular (with care) 0.5–1.0 cm.
- BL 19 *danshu shu* point of the gall bladder.

Location: 1.5 *cun* lateral to the power border of T10.
Indications:
General: eliminates heat from LI and GB, calms ST *qi*.
Particular: gall bladder disorders.
Puncture: perpendicular 0.5–1.0 cm.

- BL 20 *pishu shu* point of spleen.
Location: 1.5 *cun* lateral to the lower border of the spinous
process of T11.
Indications: regulates function of SP and eliminates damp. It
also strengthens blood.
Particular: digestive disorders, pain in the upper abdomen
and chronic diarrhoea.
Puncture: perpendicularly 0.5–1.0 cm.

- BL 21 *weishu shu* point of the stomach.
Location: 1.5 *cun* lateral to the lower border of the spinous
process of T12.
Indications:
General: dispels damp and removes stagnation.
Particular: gastric pain, gastric ulcers, nausea and chronic
diarrhoea.
Puncture: perpendicularly 0.5–1.0 cm.

- BL 22 *sanjiaoshu shu* point of the Triple Energizer.
Location: 1.5 *cun* lateral to the lower border of the spinous
process of L1.
Indications:
General: regulates movement of water in lower energizer.
Particular: local for lumbar pain, enuresis, gastralgia and
nephritis.
Puncture: perpendicularly 1–2 cm.

- BL 23 *shenshu shu* point of the kidney.
Location: 1.5 *cun* lateral to the lower border of the spinous
process of L2.
Indications:
General: eliminates damp and regulates KI *qi*.
Particular: this is a very useful point to treat in kidney *xu*
conditions. It is often used in joint and bone disorders such
as osteoarthrosis, urinary incontinence and general malaise
due to lack of kidney *qi*.
Traditionally this point should not be reduced as this drains
the *qi* of the kidney which stores the *yuan qi* for the whole
body.

Moxa can be effectively used to supply this point.
Puncture: perpendicularly 2–3 cm.
- BL 24 *quiashu*
Location: 1.5 *cun* lateral to the lower border of the spinous process of L3.
Indications:
General: strengthens *qi*.
Particular: this is the *shu* point for the lumbar spine and can be included in all treatment of back pain.
Puncture: perpendicularly 2–3 cm.
- BL 25 *dachanshu shu* point of the large intestine.
Location: 1.5 *cun* lateral to the lower border of the spinous process of L4.
Indications:
General: stimulates the function of the LI.
Particular: local for lumbar pain, sciatica, diarrhoea, constipation and abdominal distention.
Puncture: perpendicularly 2–3 cm.
- BL 26 *guanyanshu*. This is associated with *guanyan* (CV 4).
Location: 1.5 *cun* lateral to the midline, level with the lower border of the spinous process of L5.
Indications: enuresis, dysuria, abdominal distension and low back pain.
Puncture: perpendicularly 1–2 cm.
- BL 27 *xiaochangshu shu* point of the small intestine.
Location: 1.5 *cun* lateral to the midline, level with the 1st sacral foramen, in the depression between the medial border of the posterior superior iliac spine and the sacrum.
Indications: intestinal and urogenital disorders. Lumbago and sciatica.
Puncture: perpendicularly 1–2 cm. Use of moxa is effective when a supplying treatment is needed.
- BL 28 *pangguangshu shu* point of the bladder.
Location: 1.5 *cun* lateral to the midline level with the 2nd sacral foramen, in the depression between the lower medial border of the posterior inferior iliac spine and the sacrum.
Indications: Disperses *qi* of lower energizer and regulates BL function.
Particular: retention of urine, enuresis and pain in the lumbo-sacral region.
Puncture: perpendicularly 1–2 cm.

- BL 32 *ciliao*
  Location: in the second sacral foramen. This is located by identifying the first sacral foramen which lies midway between
  the spinous process of the first sacral vertebra and the
  posterior superior iliac spine, then palpating immediately
  below this point the second sacral foramen will be found.
  Indications: diseases of the urinary and reproductive systems;
  low back pain.
  Puncture: perpendicularly 2–3 cm.
- BL 39 *weiyang*
  Location: on the lateral end of the popliteal crease on the
  medial side of the tendon of biceps femoris.
  Indications: a specific point for treatment of knee joint prob-
  lems. Very effective using needle heated with moxa.
  Puncture: perpendicularly 1–2 cm.
- BL 40 *weizhong ho* point.
  Location: on the midpoint of the popliteal crease.
  Indications:
  General: Dispels damp, removes heat from blood.
  Particular: this is one of the influential points with particular
  effect on skin conditions. It is also used as the remote point
  when other bladder points are treated, thus it effects blad-
  der problems, pelvic disorders, lumbar pain and sciatica.
  Puncture: perpendicularly 2–3 cm.
- BL 55 *heyang*
  Location: 2 *cun* directly below BL 40 *weizhong*.
  Indications: sciatica and lumbago.
  Puncture: perpendicularly 2–3 cm.
- BL 57 *chengshan*
  Location: 8 *cun* below BL 40 *weizhong* and midway between
  the popliteal crease and the heel.
  Indications: sciatica, prolapse of the rectum, spasm of the
  gastrocnemius, pain in the sole of the foot and paralysis of
  the leg.
  Puncture: perpendicularly 2–3 cm.
- BL 58 *feiyang lo* point connecting with KI 4 *dazhong*.
  Location: 7 *cun* directly above BL 60 *kunlun*.
  Indications: lumbago, weakness and pain in the leg, nephritis
  and cystitis.
  Puncture: perpendicularly 2–3 cm.
- BL 60 *kunlun*
  Location: between the posterior border of the external

malleolus and medial aspect of the Achilles tendon, at the level of the tip of the malleolus.
Indications:
General: eliminates internal Wind.
Particular: sciatica, lumbago, cervical spondylosis, inflammation of the Achilles tendon, local pain in the ankle and paralysis of the leg.
Puncture: perpendicularly 1–1.5 cm.

- BL 62 *shenmai* key point for *yang chiao mai*.
Location: 0.5 *cun* directly below the external malleolus.
Indications:
General: stimulates the meridians. It is the key point of *yang chiao mai*. Used in combination with SI 3 *houxi* for autoimmune disorders, e.g. rheumatoid arthritis.
Particular: it is also sometimes effective for headache, dizziness and vertigo.
Puncture: perpendicularly 0.5–1.0 cm.

- BL 63 *jinmen xi* cleft point.
Location: anterior and inferior to BL 62 *shenmai* in a depression posterior to the tuberosity of the 5th metatarsal.
Indications: local pain, acute symptoms resulting from disturbances in the bladder organ.
Puncture: perpendicularly 0.5–1.0 cm.

- BL 65 *shugu* sedation point.
Location: posterior and inferior to the distal head of the 5th metatarsal.
Indications: headache, dizziness, lumbago and leg pain.
Puncture: perpendicularly 0.5–1.0 cm.

- BL 66 *tonggu* horory point.
Location: in the depression anterior and inferior to the 5th metatarso-phalangeal joint.
Indications: headache and dizziness. It is a useful point to tonify the BL especially during the two hours between 15.00 and 17.00 hours.
Puncture: perpendicularly 0.5 cm.

- BL 67 *zhiyin* tonification point.
Location: on the lateral side of the little toe about 0.1 *cun* posterior to the corner of the nail.
Indications: particular effect on painful labour in childbirth. It is interesting to note that in China a breach presentation of the fetus is treated with daily moxa on this point for 5 days

after which time the fetus turns to the normal head down position.

(b) Zang *organ*

Kidney KI foot *shaoyin* (Figure 3.10).

Linked with the bladder (BL).
Alarm point *mu*: GB 25 *jingmen*.
Back *shu* point: BL 23 *shenshu*.
Maximum energy time: 17.00–19.00 hours.

Together with the heart channel it forms *chao yin*, the deepest of the Six *Chiaos*.

Course
There are 27 points identified on this channel. It originates on the sole of the foot, passes along the medial aspect of the ankle, circles the medial malleolus, and ascends the medial leg to the knee. It then passes into the groin via the medial aspect of the thigh, emerging 0.5 *cun* lateral to the midine and ascends the abdomen to the thorax where it is sited 2 *cun* from the midline and terminates just below the clavicle.

Clinical applicationsm
Together with the bladder it forms the functional system, which influences the excretions of the kidney and urinary tract, also reproductive functions. It is the store for ancestral or *yuan qi*. The level of *qi* in the kidney governs the overall well-being of the individual both mentally and physically.

Use of kidney channel points is indicated in urogenital disorders, rheumatoid arthritis and depressive illness.

Most significant points
* KI 3 *taixi* source point
  Location: midway between the tip of the medial malleolus and the Achilles tendon.
  Indications:
  General: tonifies KI *qi*. Calms the Fire.
  Particular: enuresis, nephritis, cystitis, irregular menstruation.
      It is also a valuable tonification point particularly in stimulating *yin qi* of the kidney.
  Puncture: perpendicularly 1–2 cm.

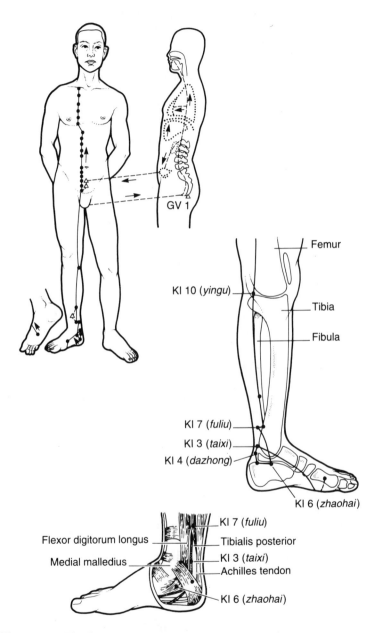

Figure 3.10 The kidney meridian (KI). The unbroken line indicates the main channel, the broken line shows internal connections.

- KI 4 *dazhong lo* point connecting with BL 64 *jinggu*.
  Location: inferior and posterior to the medial malleolus.
  Indications: point for local pain, asthma, dysuresis, constipation. It can be used to balance energy between the bladder and kidney via the *lo* meridian connecting to BL 64 *jinggu*.
  Puncture: perpendicularly 0.5–1.0 cm.
- KI 6 *zhaohai*
  Location: 1 *cun* directly below the tip of the medial malleolus.
  Indications:
  General: eliminates heat.
  Particular: dysmenorrhoea, irregular periods and local ankle problems.
  Precaution: do not use during first three months of pregnancy.
  Puncture: perpendicularly 0.5–1.0 cm.
- KI 7 *fuliu* tonification point
  Location: on the anterior border of the Achilles tendon, 2 *cun* above the medial malleolus.
  Indications:
  General: nourishes kidney *yin*, eliminates damp heat.
  Particular: cystitis, nephritis, night sweats, diarrhoea, and lumbago.
  Puncture: perpendicularly 1–2 cm.
- KI 10 *yingu ho* point
  Location: at the medial end of the popliteal crease between the tendons of semitendinosus and semimembranosus.
  Indications:
  General: tonifies KI, dispels heat and regulates lower energizer.
  Particular: knee pain. It can also be used as a remote point when other points on the kidney channel are being treated.
  Puncture: perpendicularly 1–2 cm.

3.7.5 Fire element (pericardium and triple energizer meridians)

(a) Zang *organ*

Pericardium (PC) hand *jueyin* (Figure 3.11).

Alarm point MU: CV 17 *shanzhong*

Back *shu* point: BL 14 *jueyinshu* (1.5 *cun* lateral to spinous process T4)

Maximum energy time: 19.00–21.00 hrs.

Course

There are nine points identified along this channel.

It starts 1 *cun* lateral to the nipple and then passes into the anterior aspect of the arm and descends along the midline to forearm and palm, terminating at the tip of the middle finger.

Clinical applications

The heart and pericardium together form a functional unit. In traditional Chinese medicine the heart function is associated with the brain and thought. The pericardium is primarily concerned with the circulation. It also protects and regulates cardiac function. Pericardium points have a strong effect on the circulation and are therefore indicated in circulatory and cardiac disorders.

Together with the LR channel it forms *tsui yin*, the middle of the inner three layers of the Six *Chiaos*.

Most significant points

- PC 3 *quze ho* point
  Location: the middle of the transverse cubital crease on the ulnar side of the tendon of biceps brachii.
  Indications:
  General: frees HT *qi*. Dispels heat from blood.
  Particular: gastralgia, palpitation, angina pectorus. It can be used as a remote point when other points are treated on this channel.
  Puncture: perpendicularly 1–2 cm.
- PC 4 *ximen xi* cleft point
  Location: 5 *cun* above the transverse crease of wrist, between the tendon of palmaris longus and flexor carpi radialis (Figure 3.11a).
  Indications:
  General: Calms the HT.
  Particular: this is the *xi* Cleft point and is therefore indicated in acute symptoms in this channel. Tachycardia, angina pectoris, pleuritis, and mastitis.

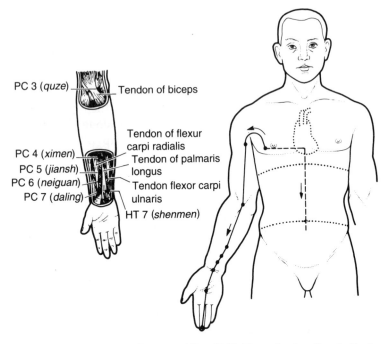

PC 3 (*quze*) — Tendon of biceps

Tendon of flexur
carpi radialis
PC 4 (*ximen*) — Tendon of palmaris
PC 5 (*jiansh*) — longus
PC 6 (*neiguan*) — Tendon flexor carpi
PC 7 (*daling*) — ulnaris
HT 7 (*shenmen*)

Figure 3.11 The pericardium meridian (PC). The unbroken line indicates the main channel, the broken line shows internal connections.

Puncture: perpendicularly 1–2 cm.

- PC 6 *neiguan lo* point connecting via transverse *lo* meridian to TE 4 *yangchi*. Key point of *yin wei mai*.
  Location: 2 *cun* proximal to the transverse wrist crease, between palmaris longus and flexor carpi radialis.
  Indications:
  General: Removes stagnation in middle energizer, regulates circulation of *qi*, calms HT and mind.
  Particular: disorders of the chest and upper abdomen including gastric and duodenal ulcers, nausea, hiccough, vomiting, heartburn. It is a useful point to give acupressure in hyperemesis.
  Puncture: perpendicular 1–2 cm.
- PC 7 *daling* source and sedative point.
  Location: On the transverse crease of the wrist, between palmaris longus and flexor carpi radialis.

Indications:
General: disperses Fire of HT, calms HT, mind and ST.
Particular: disorders of the wrist and surrounding tissues, insomnia, polyneuropathy, paralysis.
Puncture: perpendicularly 0.5–1.0 cm.

(b) Fu organ (Figure 3.12)

Triple energizer (TE) hand *chao yin*
Linked with the pericardium.

It should be noted that in Chinese this meridian is called *sanjiao* and various translations and abbreviations have been used. The term Triple Energizer has been internationally agreed in the World Health Organization, to be the current acceptable standard terminology for this meridian.

Alarm point (*mu*): CV 5 *shimen*
Back *shu* point: BL 22 *sanjiaoshu* 1.5 *cun* lateral to spinous process L1.
Maximum energy time: 21.00–23.00 hrs.

Course
There are 23 points identified along the course of this channel. It starts on the ulnar corner of the little finger nail, ascends the posterior aspect of the forearm and arm, passes over the shoulder and lateral side of the neck and terminates at the lateral corner of the eye.

Clinical application
The Triple Energizer controls three areas of function. The upper energizer is responsible for the intake of *qi* and influences the area lying above the diaphragm including the heart and lungs; the middle energizer is responsible for digestive function and influences the abdomen and includes the stomach, spleen and gall bladder organs; the lower energizer is responsible for excretion and influences the pelvic area and includes the small intestine, large intestine, liver, kidney, bladder organs and the uterus.

Together with the GB it forms *chao yang*, the middle of the outer three of the Six *Chiaos*.

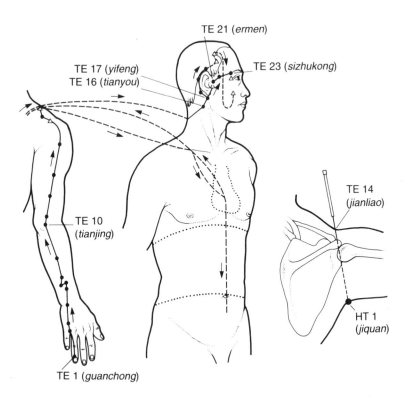

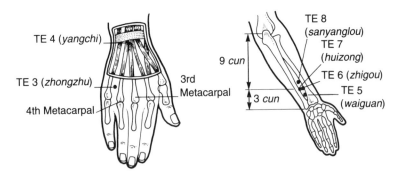

Figure 3.12 The Triple Energizer (TE). The unbroken line indicates the main channel, the broken line shows internal connections.

Most significant points

- TE 1 *guanchong tsing* point
  Location: on the ulnar side of the ring finger 0.1 *cun* posterior to the corner of the nail (Figure 3.12).
  Indications:
  General: eliminates heat.
  Particular: headache, inflamed eyes, sore throat.
  Puncture: obliquely 0.3 cm.

- TE 3 *zhongzhu* tonification point
  Location: on the posterior aspect of the hand, between the 4th and 5th metacarpals and proximal to the metacarpophalangeal joint.
  Indications:
  General: tonifies and regulates *qi*.
  Particular: ear disorders, local painful conditions, polyneuropathy of the hand, headaches.
  Puncture: perpendicularly 1–2 cm.

- TE 4 *yangchi* source point
  Location: in a depression of the transverse crease of the dorsum of wrist between extensor digitorum longus and extensor minimi digiti (Figure 3.12).
  Indications:
  General: eliminates heat, relaxes the tendons, removes obstuctions from the meridian and its collaterals. Stimulates *qi* in the TE meridian.
  Particular: disorders of the wrist joint and surrounding tissues.
  Puncture: perpendicularly 0.5–1.0 cm.

- TE 5 *waiguan lo* point connecting to PC 7 *daling*
  Location: at midpoint of the ulna and radius, 2 *cun* proximal to the wrist (Figure 3.12).
  Indications:
  General: it is the key point of *yang wei mai* and, with GB 41 (foot *linqi*), the key point of *dai mai*, is used to relieve external symptoms.
  Particular: torticollis, temporal headache, pain and polyneuropathy of the arm, arthritis of the wrist. Can also affect disorders on the PC channel through the *lo* point connection to PC.
  Puncture: perpendicularly 1–2 cm.

gou horory point
: between the ulna and radius 3 *cun* proximal to the
Figure 3.12).
indications:
General: disperses stagnant blood and regulates the *zang
fu.*
Particular: constipation, irritable bowel disease. Stimulation
of *qi* within the TE meridian.
Puncture: perpendicularly 1–2 cm.

- TE 7 *huizong xi* cleft point
Location: 1 finger width lateral to TE 6 *zhigou* on the radial
side of the ulna (Figure 3.12).
Indications:
General: deafness.
Particular: pain in the upper extremities, acute symptoms of
the TE.
Puncture: perpendicularly 1–2 cm.

- TE 8 *sanyanglou* connection of 3 *yang* meridians
Location: between the ulna and radius, 4 *cun* proximal to the
wrist (Figure 3.12).
Indications:
General: pain in the chest wall, intercostal neuralgia, herpes
zosta.
Particular: pain in the arm, sudden deafness, aphasia.
Puncture: perpendicularly 1–2 cm.

- TE 10 *tianying ho* point and sedation point
Location: 1 *cun* posterior and superior to the olecranon, in the
depression made by flexing the elbow (Figure 3.12).
Indications:
General: removes obstructions from the meridians and their
collaterals.
Particular: disorders of the elbow joint and surrounding tis-
sue, unilateral headaches.
Puncture: perpendicularly 1–2 cm.

- TE 14 *jianliao*
Location: the point lies between the acromion and the greater
tubercle of the humerus when the arm is held by the side
(Figure 3.12).
Indications:
General: stimulates blood circulation, reduces pain.
Particular: disorders of the shoulder joint, pain in the arm,

paralysis in the arm.

Puncture: perpendicularly towards HT 1 *jiquan* 2–3 cm.

- TE 16 *tianyou*

Location: posterior and inferior to the mastoid process, on the posterior border of the sterno-cleido-mastoid, at the level of the angle of the jaw (Figure 3.12).

Indication: It is interesting to note that when mobilizing the apophyseal joint of C2 using a Maitland technique, there is direct pressure on this acupoint. The symptoms presented when the second cervical nerve is affected include reduction of mobility, hemispherical headache with eye pain and tinnitus. These symptoms are similar to those listed in the Chinese literature that are affected by treating this acupoint.

Puncture: perpendicularly 2–3 cm.

- TE 17 *yifeng*

Location: in the depression posterior to the ear lobe and anterior to the mastoid process (Figure 3.12).

Indications:

General: it is the crossing point of the GB and TE and has the effect of eliminating Wind.

Particular: deafness, tinnitus, parotitis and facial paralysis.

Puncture: this point can be pierced to 2–3 cm if the needle is directed anterior and upward, otherwise needle 1–2 cm. NB In current practice in China it is often injected with vitamin B12 in cases of facial palsy.

- TE 21 *ermen*

Location: when the mouth is open, in the depression in front of the intertragic notch and slightly superior to the condyloid head of the mandible (Figure 3.12).

Indications:

General: benefits the brain.

Particular: deafness, tinnitus, otitis media, facial palsy and disorders of the mandible.

Puncture: perpendicularly 1–2 cm with patient's mouth slightly open.

TE 23 *sizhukong*

Location: on the lateral border of the orbit at the lateral tip of the eyebrow (Figure 3.12).

Indications: headache, eye disorders.

Puncture: horizontally and posteriorly 1–2 cm.

3.7.6 Wood element (gall bladder and liver meridians)

Tissue: muscle and tendon
Sense organ: eye
Sense: sight

(a) Fu *organ*

Gall bladder (GB) (Figure 3.13).

Linked with the liver (LR)
Alarm point (*mu*): GB 24 *riyue* (7th intercostal space)
Back *shu* point: BL 19 *danshu* (1.5 *cun* lateral to spinous process
  T10).
Maximum energy time: 23.00–1.00 hrs.

Course
There are 44 points identified along the course of this channel. It starts at the corner of the eye and passes down to the tragus, ascends to circumvent the ear then descends to the occiput. It passes back over the head to the middle of the forehead, retraces its path more medially and descends to the occiput once more, passing over the shoulder into the lateral aspect of the thorax and abdomen. It then descends the lateral aspect of the thigh, leg and foot to end at the lateral side of the 4th toenail.

Clinical applications
There is a close relationship with the liver in the function of this channel. They both have an influence on the circulation of vital energy throughout the body. The gall bladder is a very useful channel in treating headache and migraine. It is also effective in muscular disorders, particularly in the neck and shoulders.

The leg points are used both for local musculo-skeletal problems, as well as distal points for liver and gall bladder dysfunction.

It is linked with the TE channel to form *chao yang*, which is the middle of the outer three of the Six *Chiaos*.

Most significant points
* GB 1 *tongziliao*
  Location: 0.5 *cun* lateral to the outer canthus (Figure 3.13).

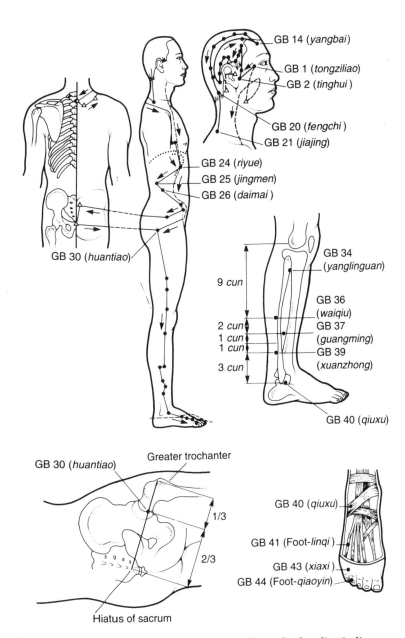

Figure 3.13 The gall bladder meridian (GB). The unbroken line indicates the main channel, the broken line shows internal connections.

Indications: eye disorders, frontal and occipital headache, trigeminal neuralgia.

NB As this is an end point GB 44 foot *qiaoyin* can be effective as a distal point in treating local pain.

Puncture: obliquely 1–2 cm horizontally and laterally.

- GB 2 *tinghui*

  Location: in a depression when the mouth is opened just behind the condyle of the mandible (Figure 3.13).

  Indications:

  General: eliminates Wind and promotes auditory function.

  Particular: deafness, tinnitus, otitis media, local TMJ joint problems.

  Puncture: perpendicularly 1–2 cm.

- GB 14 *yangbai*

  Location: 1 *cun* above the midpoint of the eyebrow (Figure 3.13).

  Indication:

  General : eliminates Wind, relief of pain and muscle spasms.

  Particular: eye disorders, frontal headache, migraine and trigeminal neuralgia.

  Puncture: horizontally 1–2 cm either towards eyebrow or hairline.

- GB 20 *fengchi*

  Location: between the origins of sterno-cleido-mastoid and trapezius (Figure 3.13).

  Indications: this is a coalescent of GB and *yang wei mai*. It eliminates Wind and heat, promotes *qi* and blood and removes obstructions from the meridian.

  Particular: torticollis, vertigo, cervical pain, occipital headache, hypertension.

  Puncture: perpendicularly towards opposite eye 2–3 cm. NB this point should not be needled too deeply!

- GB 21 *jianjing* (It is an additional alarm point of the gall bladder).

  Location: midway between GV 14 *dazhui* and the acromion process at the highest point of the shoulder. The angle of the first rib can be palpated immediately below this point (Figure 3.13).

  Indications: pain in the shoulder and back, stiff neck, disorders of liver and gall bladder.

  This point can be treated with a downward pressure using the thumb. Pressure is rythmically continued until the patient feels no pain although the initial application of pressure is very uncomfortable. This is a technique widely used by physiotherapists who are trained in Maitland mobilizing techniques and is highly effective to promote relief of muscle tension in the neck and shoulders.

Puncture: perpendicular 1–2 cm. NB This point should be needled with care as the apex of the lung lies immediately below.

- GB 24 *riyue* alarm (*mu*) point of the gall bladder.
  Location: on the nipple line in the 7th intercostal space (Figure 3.13).
  Indications: liver disorders, hepatitis, cholecystitis, gastritis and hiccough. Puncture: obliquely 1–2 cm. NB A careful technique is necessary to avoid piercing the pleura.
- GB 25 *jingmen* alarm (*mu*) point of the kidney.
  Location: At the lower border of the free end of the 12th rib (Figure 3.13).
  Indications:
  General: disorders of liver and gall bladder.
  Particular: intercostal neuralgia; in kidney deficiency syndromes it can be heated with moxa along with BL 23 *shenshu* (back *shu* point of kidney).
  Puncture: perpendicular 0.5–1.0 cm.
- GB 26 *daimai*
  Location: midway between the free ends of the 11th and 12th ribs level with the umbilicus (Figure 3.13).
  Indications:
  General: disorders of liver and gall bladder.
  Particular: lumbago, intercostal and abdominal pain, amenorrhoea and irregular menstruation.
  Puncture: perpendicularly 2–3 cm.
- GB 30 *huantiao*
  Location: at the junction of the middle and lateral third of a line drawn from the upper border of the greater trochanter and the hiatus of the sacrum (Figure 3.13).
  Indication: it is the coalescent point of the GB and BL meridians and affects the strength of the back and lower extremities, eliminates cold and Wind, invigorates *qi* and removes obstructions.
  Particular: sciatica, low back pain, paralysis, polyneuropathy

of the leg, disorders of the hip joint and its surrounding
tissue.
Puncture: perpendicularly 3–6 cm. This variation of depth is
due to the varying thickness of adipose tissue overlying the
muscle.

* GB 34 *yanglinguan ho* point. Influential for muscles and
tendons.
Location: in the depression anterior and inferior to the head
of fibula (Figure 3.13).
Indications:
General: influential point for tendons and affects the function
of the gall bladder organ specifically. This point can be used
to reinforce treatment for muscles/tendons anywhere in the
body, e.g. local points would be used for tennis elbow and
GB 34 as a distal influential point.
Particular: disorders of the knee and paralysis. It can be combined with LI 4 (*hegu*) and LR 3 (*taichong*) to give deep
relaxation if the patient is agitated.
Puncture: perpendicularly 2–3 cm or downward and anterior
with strong stimulation in paralysis.

* GB 36 *waiqui xi* cleft point
Location: 7 *cun* above the tip of the lateral malleolus on the
posterior border of the fibula (Figure 3.13).
Indication: pain in the lateral aspect of the leg. It is the *xi* cleft
point and can be used for acute situations in the gall bladder
channel.
Puncture: perpendicularly 2–3 cm.

* GB 37 *guangming, lo* point connecting to LR 3 *taichong*.
Location: 5 *cun* proximal to the lateral malleolus and on the
anterior border of the fibula (Figure 3.13).
Indications:
General: disorders of liver and gall bladder, eye problems.
Particular: local leg pain.
Puncture: perpendicularly 1–3 cm.

* GB 39 *xuanzhong*, influential point for marrow (brain and
nervous system in TCM).
Location: 3 *cun* above the lateral malleolus, between the pos-
terior border of the fibula and peroneus longus and brevis
(Figure 3.13).
Indications:
General: it is one of the Eight Influential Points asso-

ciated with marrow. It stimulates circulation of blood and eliminates Wind.
Particular: important distal point for torticollis, paralysis of the leg, local soft tissue problems.
Puncture: perpendicularly 1–2 cm.

- GB 40 *qiuxu* source point connecting with LR 5 *ligou* (via transverse *lo* meridian).
Location: anterior and inferior to the lateral malleolus, in the depression on the lateral side of the tendon of extensor digitorum longus (Figure 3.13).
Indications: ankle joint problems, chest pain and general leg pain.
Puncture: perpendicularly 1–2 cm.

- GB 41 foot *linqi* horary point. Key point or *dai mai*.
Location: in the depression anterior to the base of the 4th and 5th metatarsal bones (Figure 3.13).
Indications:
General: reduces Fire and relieves pain.
Particular: headaches and local joint problems.
Puncture: perpendicularly 1–2 cm.

- GB 43 *xiaxi* tonification point
Location: on the cleft between the 4th and 5th metatarsal bones, 0.5 *cun* proximal to the margin of the web (Figure 3.13).
Indications: deafness, headache, dizziness, chest pain, intercostal neuralgia.
Puncture: perpendicularly 0.5–1.0 cm.

- GB 44 foot *qiaoyin*
Location: on the lateral side of the tip of the 4th toe, 0.1 *cun* lateral to the corner of the nail (Figure 3.13).
Indications: headache (used as end point with GB 1 *tongziliao*).
Puncture: perpendicularly 0.2 cm.

(b) Zang organ

Liver (LR) linked with gall bladder (Figure 3.14)
Alarm point (*mu*): LR 14 *qimen*
Back *shu* point: BL 18 *ganshu* (1.5 *cun* lateral to the spinous process of T9).
Maximum energy time: 1.00–3.00 hrs.

Course
There are 14 points identified along the course of this channel. It
starts at the lateral corner of the hallux, passes along the medial
side of the foot, leg and thigh to the external genitalia. It then
ascends the abdomen to end at the 6th intercostal space on the
lateral chest wall.

Clinical applications
The liver channel is closely associated with the genitalia and
their functions. The distal points are indicated in urogenital
functions, eye disorders, headaches, liver and gall bladder disorders. The trunk points are used in cholecystitis and metabolic
disorders.
    Together with the PC channel it forms *Tsui Yin*, which is the *yin*
hinge of the Six *Chiaos*.

Most significant points

• LR 2 *xingjian* sedation point
    Location: 0.5 *cun* proximal to the margin of the web between
       the first and second toes (Figure 3.14b).
    Indications:
    General: soothes the liver and regulates *qi* circulation.
    Particular: redness and swelling of the eye, intercostal pain,
       urethritis, enuresis and insomnia.
    Puncture: obliquely 0.5–1.0 cm.
• LR 3 *taichong* source point connecting to GB 37 *guangming* (via
    the transverse *lo* meridian).
    Location: 2 *cun* proximal to the margin of the web between
       the 1st and 2nd toes (Figure 3.14b).
    Indications:
    General: Soothes the liver, promotes *qi* and blood and regu-
       lates menstrual flow.
    Particular: headache, inflammation of the eye, head and chest
       pain. With LI 4 (*hegu*) it forms a powerful combination to
       reduce agitation and alleviate insomnia. NB This point can
       reduce blood pressure and should be used cautiously in
       patients with blood pressure problems.
    Puncture: perpendicularly 1–2 cm or 1–2 cm obliquely
       upward.

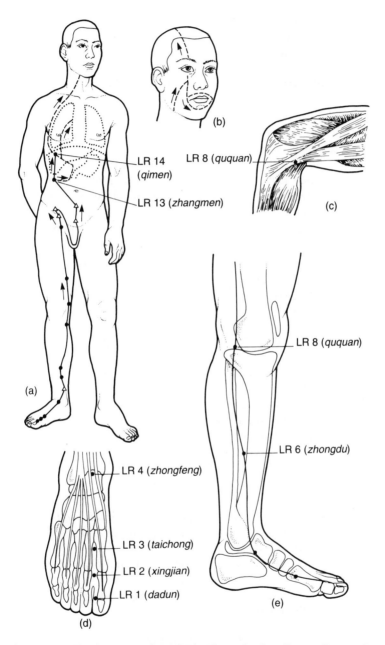

Figure 3.14 The liver meridian (LR). The unbroken line indicates the main channel, the broken line shows internal connections.

- LR 6 *zhongdu xi* cleft point
  Location: 7 *cun* superior to the tip of the medial malleolus, on
    the posterior border of the tibia (Figure 3.14c).
  Indications:
  General: acute symptoms of the liver channel, abdominal
    pain and diarrhoea.
  Particular: pain in the lower extremities.
  Puncture: perpendicularly or obliquely 1–2 cm.
- LR 8 *ququan ho* point
  Location: At the medial end of the transverse crease of
    the knee joint, in a depression at the anterior border of
    semimembranosus and semitendinosus (Figure 3.14d).
  Indications:
  General: eliminates damp and heat from the lower energizer.
  Particular: disorders of the knee (moxa is effective), dys-
    menorrhoea, urogenital infections. It is an influential point
    for lower extremity pain.
  Puncture: perpendicularly 2–3 cm.
- LR 13 *zhangmen mu* point of the spleen; influential point of the
  zang organs.
  Location: on the free end of the 11th rib (Figure 3.14a).
  Indications:
  General: soothes the liver, regulates *qi*, stimulates blood
    circulation.
  Particular: disorders of liver and gall bladder, abdominal dis-
    tension, pain in the costal region.
  Puncture: perpendicularly 1–2 cm.
- LR 14 *qimen mu* point of the liver.
  Location: On the mamillary line in the 6th intercostal space
    (Figure 3.14a).
  Indications:
  General: it is the coalescent point of LR, SP and *yin wei mai*
    meridian. It soothes the liver, regulates *qi* and resolves co-
    agulation of blood.
  Particular: pain of the upper abdomen and chest, bronchial
    asthma, intercostal neuralgia.
  Puncture: obliquely 0.5–1.0 cm with great care to avoid punc-
    turing the pleura.

3.7.7 Conclusion

It is interesting to note that those physiotherapists who use mobi-
lizing/manipulative techniques will be able to identify many

acupoints which are located over joints which are treated in musculo-skeletal disorders. The bladder back *shu* points on the back are a good example.

3.8 THE EIGHT EXTRA MERIDIANS

These meridians do not have a governing organ as do the main 'master meridians' and they do not have a specific place in the Five Elements. Two of them, Conception and Governor, have their own points, whereas the other six utilize points on the main channels. They do, however, have a relationship to body functions:

1. the brain and spinal cord, and hormonal control;
2. the musculo-skeletal system;
3. the genitalia;
4. the circulatory system and formation of blood cells;
5. the hepatic and bilary systems (Low, 1983).

The eight extra meridians are described below. They will be considered individually and the various connections with other meridians briefly described. The use of paired meridians will then be addressed.

3.8.1 *Du mai* (Figure 3.15)

It is confusing that this meridian is called *du mai* indicating its position as one of the eight extra meridians and in some texts the code DU is used to describe the points on this channel. The most recent World Health Organization standard coding however is GV, short for Governing Vessel, which is a translation of the Chinese.

Course
It commences in the right kidney, passes to CV 1, ascends the midline of the spinal column, passing over the head to end at GV 28 which lies between the upper lip and the gum.

Clinical applications
Various points on this channel have important connections with other organs and meridians as well as having local therapeutic effects. It governs the six *yang* channels and has a general co-ordinating function for the regions of the body and the organs.

Excessive *yang* energy causes blocking of *qi* which results in stiffness of the spine and sometimes headaches and eye pain. Conversely, too little *yang* energy in *du mai* results in a sagging posture.

The association with the pelvis can be influential on haemorrhoids and urogenital disorders.

It should be noted that those points on *du mai* that are level with the bladder points which are lying contralaterally to the spine, also have some influence on the organs associated with the bladder or back *shu* points, e.g. GV 4 is level with BL 23 (back *shu*) point of the kidney organ.

This strong connection with the kidneys means that this meridian is of importance when formulating a treatment programme for arthritic conditions.

It can also be considered when faced with the diagnosis of myalgic encephalomyelitis (ME or post viral syndrome). This results when pathogenic factors are not completely expelled. In these cases GV 13 (*taodao*) and GV 14 (*dazhui*) are indicated (Maciocia, 1989).

Most significant points

- GV 1 *changqiang* reunion point with *ren mai* and the kidneys.
  Location: midway between the tip of the coccyx and the anus, located prone.
  Indications: haemorrhoids (moxa is effective), coccydynia, prolapse of the rectum.
  Puncture: 0.5–1.0 cm obliquely or 1–2 cm horizontally.
- GV 4 *mingmen*
  Location: between the spinous processes of L2 and L3.
  Indications: lumbago, urogenital disorders, sciatica. (Moxa can be effective on this point.)
  Puncture: 1–2 cm with needle inserted in upward direction.
- GV 13 *taodao* reunion point with the bladder meridian.
  Location: below the spinous process of T1.
  Indications: stiffness of back, occipital headache, cervical spondylosis.
  Puncture: obliquely upward 1–2 cm.
- GV 14 *daizui* reunion point for all the *yang* meridians.
  Location: below the spinous process of C7.
  Indications: asthma, eczema, immune enhancing effect,

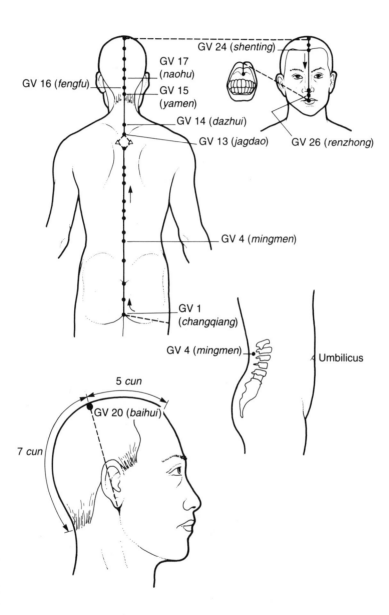

Figure 3.15 *Du mai* (GV). The unbroken line indicates the main meridian, the broken line shows internal connections.

depression, occipital headache, cervical sponylosis, torticollis.
Puncture: perpendicularly 1–2 cm.

- GV 15 *yamen* union with *yang wei*.
Location: 0.5 *cun* above hairline, between the spinous process of C1 and C2.
Indications: stiff neck, occipital headache, neurosis.
Puncture: perpendicularly with head slightly flexed, directed towards mandible 1–2 cm.

- GV 16 *fengfu* union with *yang wei* and bladder meridian.
Location: directly below the occipital protuberance, in the midline 1 *cun* above the hairline.
Indications: headache, stiffness in the upper cervical spine when combined with BL 10 *tianshu*.
Puncture: perpendicularly 1–1.5 cm.

- GV 17 *naohu* union with bladder meridian.
Location: 1.5 *cun* directly above GV 16 *fengfu*.
Indications: headache, stiffness and pain in the neck.
Puncture: obliquely 1–1.5 cm.

- GV 20 *baihui* reunion point for all *yang* meridians.
Location: it lies 5 *cun* behind the anterior hairline and 7 *cun* above posterior hairline and where the midline is crossed by a line joining the highest points of the ears.
Indications: it has the action of summoning energy to the head. Therefore it should not be tonified when the patient is hypertensive. It can be effective in raising *qi* when central *qi* is weak, with symptoms such as prolapsed uterus or bladder.
Treatment note: moxa applied at this point and at GV 1 *changqiang* can be very effective for haemorrhoids.

- GV 24 *shenting* reunion point for stomach and bladder meridians.
Location: 0.5 *cun* above the midpoint of the anterior line.
Indications: frontal headache, rhinitis.
Puncture: obliquely 1–1.5 cm.

- GV 26 *renzhong* reunion point with the bladder and stomach meridians.
Location: in the midline at the junction of the upper and lower two thirds of the upper lip.
Indications: it is effective for acute situations, e.g. acute lumbago.
Puncture: 0.5–1–0 cm with point tilted upwards.

The key point for *du mai* is SI 3 which is on the crease made by the 5th MCP joint of the hand. It may seem rather strange that this seemingly unconnected point can open the activity of *du mai*. It is hypothesized that *du mai* has a strong influence on and focuses all the *yang* energy in the body. *Yang* energy is also primarily superficial and if related back to the outer layer or most *yang* layer of the Six *Chiaos*, this gives a connection to the small intestine meridian through ascending energy and thus to the *yu* point or SI 3 (*houxi*). It is as you can see a rather tortuous connection.

3.8.2 *Ren mai* (Figure 3.16)

Course
It starts in the pelvic cavity and emerges at the perineum and runs up the midline to the neck and lower jaw to the centre of the mental labial groove. It passes around the mouth and passes through ST 4 (*dicang*) bilaterally entering the eyes at ST 1 (*chengqi*).

Clinical applications
Ren mai controls the six *yin* channels and the anterior aspect of the body. It regulates the energy of the reproductive system and after the menopause tonifies blood and *yin* to reduce the effects of kidney *yin* syndromes, e.g. night sweats and hot flushes. Because of its strong association with reproductive function it is also called the Conception Vessel (CV). The latter name is adopted in reference to this meridian when identifying points.

It influences the energy in all three parts of the Triple Energizer meridian and can therefore affect chronic respiratory disorders, e.g. asthma as well as *qi* in the abdomen and the distribution of body fluids.

It is interesting to note that abdominal incisions made along the midline cut through some vital points on the CV meridian and it could be argued that this may cause more post-operative debility than a transverse incision.

Particular symptoms to look out for which could be influenced by *ren mai*, with the most effective points, are:

- Urinary infections and other disturbances: CV 2 *qugu* and CV 3 *zhongji*.
- Genital disturbances: CV 3 *zhongji* and CV 4 *guanyuan*.

- Lack of vitality/energy: CV 6 *qihai*.
- General weakness: CV 8 *shenjue*.
- Fluid regulation and oedema: CV 9 *shuifen*.
- Gastric disturbances: CV 12 *zhongwan*.
- Lung problems: CV 17 *shanzhong*.
- Brachial spasm: CV 22 *tiantu*.

Most significant points

- CV 2 *qugu* connecting with SP, KI, LR.
  Location: on the midline of the upper border of symphysis pubis.
  Indications: urogenital disorders, e.g. retention or incontinence of urine.
  Puncture: perpendicularly 2–4 cm.
- CV 3 *zhongji mu* point of BL; connecting with the tendino-muscular meridians of LR SP ST KI.
  Location: 4 *cun* below the umbilicus.
  Indications: urogenital disorders, cystitis, enuresis. A good point to heat with Moxa.
  Puncture: perpendicularly 2–4 cm.
- CV 4 *guanyuan mu* point of SI; connecting with *chong mai* and SP, KI, LR.
  Location: on the midline 3 *cun* below the umbilicus.
  Indications: urogenital disorders, dysmenorrhoea, cystitis, enuresis. A good point to heat with Moxa.
  Puncture: perpendicularly 2–4 cm.
- CV 6 *qihai*
  Location: on the midline 1.5 *cun* below the umbilicus.
  Indications: this is an important point to treat when there is general weakness. Combined with ST 36 *zusanli* and SP 6 *sanyinjiao* it is effective in chronic fatigue and hypotension, when the points are heated with Moxa.
  Puncture: perpendicularly 2–4 cm.
- CV 7 *yinjiao mu* point of lower energizer; connected with *chong mai* and KI.
  Location: 1 *cun* below the umbilicus on the midline.
  Indications: urethritis, endometritis, irregular menstruation, post-partum pain, pruritus vulvae, hernia.
  Puncture: perpendicularly 2–4 cm.

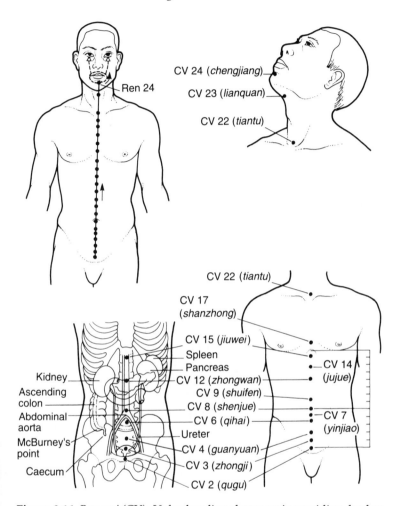

Figure 3.16 *Ren mai* (CV). Unbroken line shows main meridian, broken line shows internal connections.

- CV 8 *shenjue*
  Location: umbilicus
  Indications: general weakness. Use Moxa as needling is forbidden. One method of heating this point is to fill the umbilicus with salt and burn cones of Moxa on top of it.
- CV 9 *shuifen*
  Location: 1 *cun* above the umbilicus on the midline.

Indications: influential point for fluid balance in the body. Effective point for oedema when treated in combination with LU 7 *lieque* and KI 6 *zhaohai* using Moxa.

Puncture: perpendicular 2–4 cm.

- CV 12 *zhongwan mu* point of the middle energizer and the ST; connected to SI.

  Location: on the midline midway between the umbilicus and xiphoid process, 4 *cun* above the umbilicus.

  Indications: gastric and duodenal ulcers, nausea, digestive problems, abdominal distension and liver disorders.

  Puncture: perpendicularly 2–4 cm.

- CV 14 *jujue mu* point of HT

  Location: on the midline 6 *cun* above the umbilicus.

  Indications: stomach disorders, palpitations, mental disturbances such as insomnia and agitation.

  Puncture: 2 cm obliquely downward.

- CV 15 *jiuwei lo* point and connects with *chong mai*.

  Location: 7 *cun* above umbilicus.

  Indications: pain in the cardiac region, gastralgia, vomiting.

  Puncture: 1–2 cm obliquely downward.

- CV 17 *Shanzhong mu* point of upper energizer and PC; it connects with LU, PC, KI, SP, SI. It connects with the tendino muscular meridians of the PC LU and HT.

  Location: on the sternum on a level with the nipples at the level of the 4th intercostal space.

  Indications: heart and lung disorders, bronchial asthma disorders of the chest wall.

  Treatment note: this is an effective point to apply acupressure in cases where patients are unable to produce sputum.

  Puncture: 1–2 cm horizontally directed either sideways upwards or downwards.

- CV 22 *tiantu* connecting with *yin wei*.

  Location: at the centre of the supra-sternal fossa 0.5 *cun* above the sternal notch.

  Indications: bronchial asthma, pharyngitis, hiccough. It is also sited close to the thyroid gland and is believed to influence the production of thyroxine when treated.

  Puncture: this is a point which needs to be very carefully pierced as it lies near to the great vessels and other vital organs in the mediastinum.

Method: perpendicularly 0.3–0.8 cm then directed downwards along the posterior border of the sternum 2–3 cm.

- CV 23 *lianquan*
  Location: midway between the upper border of the cricoid cartilage and the lower border of the mandible.
  Indications: aphasia, pharyngitis, laryngitis.
  Puncture: obliquely towards base of tongue 2–3 cm.
- CV 24 *jengjiang* connecting with LR, GV, ST.
  Location: at the depression in the middle of the labial groove.
  Indications: facial paralysis, toothache.
  Puncture: perpendicularly 0.5–1.0 cm.

The key point is LU 7 (*lieque*). This is the *lo* point of the lungs. Following through the Six *Chiaos* the energy of this *yin* meridian flows to the interior when it reaches *yang ming*. From there it gets diverted to *tai yin*, which ascends from SP 1 to LI 11 towards its terminal point and at LU 7 (*lieque*) it counters the *yang* energy from *yang ming* and thus this point becomes the means of tapping into the *ren mai* meridian.

3.8.3 *Chong mai* (Figure 3.17)

This is a very complex meridian having many different functions at different levels. Together with *ren mai* it regulates the uterus and menstruation and nourishes blood.

This meridian is believed to have its source in the kidneys where it then descends (via the uterus in the female) and emerges at CV 1 (*huiyin*). It then ascends via CV 4 (*guanyuan*) entering into the kidney meridian at KI 11 (*henggu*), thence to KI 21 (*youmen*) distributing energy to the organs and viscera *en route*.

Symptoms which could be the result of a disturbance in *chong mai* are: pain and fullness in the chest region; digestive symptoms, e.g. poor appetite and abdominal distension; menstrual disturbances where moving of *qi* and blood is required.

Its key point is SP 4 (*gongsun*). This point is derived in a similar way to that of *ren mai*. The energy enters *tai yin* but this time descends to the foot and at SP 4, the *lo* point of spleen, it meets the opposing energy of *yang ming*.

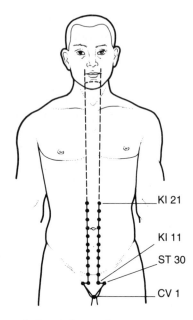

Figure 3.17 *Chong mai*, the vital vessel.

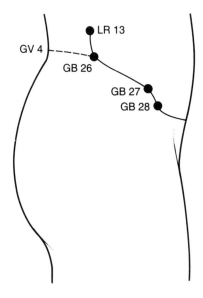

Figure 3.18 *Dai mai*, the girdle vessel.

3.8.4 *Dai mai* (Figure 3.18)

This meridian girdles the abdomen connecting all the meridians which ascend and descend the trunk. It derives its energy from the gall bladder and liver meridians and receives *yuan qi* (ancestral energy) which originates from the kidneys.

It can be seen, by the very nature of its position, that it is of importance in the function of all the meridians it connects.

Symptoms which may originate from disturbances in this meridian are:

* all female problems, e.g. dysmenorrhoea;
* acute pain in the lumbar region;
* muscular disturbances (NB the influence of gall bladder meridian);
* headaches especially when combined with menstrual problems, the reason being that energy can get 'stuck' below this meridian as it girdles the abdomen thus causing symptoms below in the uterus and above in the upper portions of the gall bladder and liver meridians;
* this meridian girdles the meridians of the legs and any disturbance in it could affect the circulation, resulting in coldness of the limbs.

Its key point is GB 41 (*zulinqi*). This is the Wood (*yu*) point of the gall bladder with which *dai mai* has strong links.

3.8.5 *Yang chiao mai* (Figure 3.19)

This may be regarded as a branch of the bladder meridian and is responsible for the transport of *yang* energy. Its greatest influence is mostly in the head. It forms a pair with *yin chiao mai* which is a branch of the kidney meridian and transports *yin* energy. Together they influence the state of the eyes.

Course

It starts in the region of the lateral malleolus ascending through BL 62 (*shenmai*), BL 61 (*pushen*), BL 59 (*fuyang*), to GB 29 (femur *juliao*). It then winds around the shoulder to SI 10 (*naoshu*), LI 14 (*binao*), LI 15 (*jianyu*), LI 16 (*jugu*). It then enters the face and connects ST 4 (*dicang*), ST 3 (*juliao*), ST 1 (*chengqi*), thence to BL 1 (*jingming*). There is then an extra connection over the head to GV 20 (*baihui*).

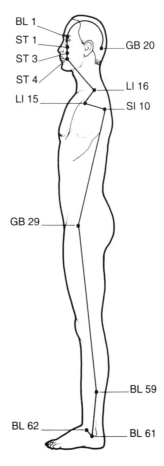

Figure 3.19 *Yang chiao mai* (*yang* heel vessel).

Symptoms which may be influenced by this meridian:

- If there is too much *yang* the eyes have difficulty closing which results in insomnia.
- Wind symptoms causing stiff neck, headache, rhinitis. NB In the combination of a stiff neck and headache this meridian can be very effective.
- Low back pain which is acute and unilateral following the bladder channel line.

- Hot and inflamed joints, as in rheumatoid arthritis. Abscess formation. Pains in the renal area. Stiffness where perverse energy has invaded the meridian which could be anywhere in the region of the meridian pathway, e.g. outer leg, coccydynia, dryness of eyes.

Its key point is BL 62 (*shenmai*). This is the point where descending ancestral energy meets with rising energy of *yang chiao mai* and leaves the vessel.

3.8.6 *Yin chiao mai* (Figure 3.20)

This is considered a secondary vessel of the kidney meridian. Its main sphere of influence is on the lower abdomen and the eyes.

Course
It runs up the medial aspect of the leg from KI 2 (Rangu) through KI 6 (*zhaohai*) KI 8 (*jiaoxin*) to the inguinal ligament where it goes deep into the abdomen, ascending until it emerges at the clavicular region, connecting with *yang chiao mai* at BL 1 (*jingming*).

Symptoms which may arise from this meridian
It is associated with pregnancy and childbirth, also fluid balance. When the whole pathway is affected with excess of *yin*, the joints in all the limbs become stiff and the muscles tight and painful in the trunk and neck. If the lower part is affected it leads to coldness in the legs and possible phlebitis.

If there is a lack of *yin* energy and therefore an excess of *yang*, pain may be experienced in the medial leg and low abdomen. In the higher part where *yin chiao mai* passes through the chest, there could be difficulty in breathing and a feeling of constriction in the chest. When there is excess of *yin* the eyelids feel very heavy and the patient feels sleepy, which is contrary to when there is too much *yang* and insomnia results. Thus treatment of eye problems may well involve the balance of *yang chiao mai* and *yin chiao mai*.

The key point is KI 6 (*zhaohai*). This vessel is considered to be the secondary vessel of the kidney and KI 6 the point where ancestral energy enters the meridian.

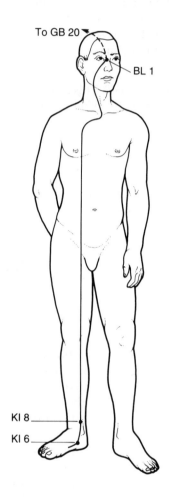

Figure 3.20 *Yin chiao mai* (*yin* heel vessel).

3.8.7 *Yang wei mai* (Figure 3.21)

This can also be considered a secondary vessel to the bladder meridian, but as its' name suggests, it is concerned with superficial *wei qi*. It is connected with the two most superficial chiaos *tai yang* and *shao yang*, through the gall bladder and bladder meridians.

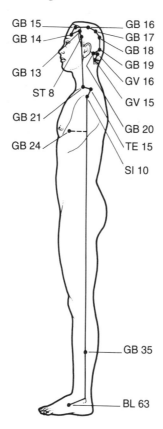

GB 15
GB 14
GB 13
ST 8
GB 21
GB 24

GB 16
GB 17
GB 18
GB 19
GV 16
GV 15
GB 20
TE 15
SI 10

GB 35

BL 63

Figure 3.21 *Yang wei mai* (*yang* regulating vessel).

Course

It starts at BL 63 (*yinmen*) and ascends the lateral aspect of the leg through GB 35 (*yangjiao*), the lateral area of the abdomen and chest to SI 10 (*naoshu*). It then travels up to the face ST 8 (*touwei*) via TH 15 (*tianliao*) GB 21 (*jiangjing*), then into the gall bladder meridian at GB 13 (*benshen*), GB 14 (*yangbai*), GB 15 (head *linqi*), passing over the head to GB 20 (*fengchi*) thence to GV 16 (*fengfu*) and ends at GV 15 (*yamen*).

It can be seen that there are strong connections with the gall bladder as well as the stomach, small intestine, Triple Energizer and governor meridians. It is responsible for the regulation of protective *wei qi* by uniting the *yang* meridians. It also has a significance in the system of the Six *Chiaos*, namely *tai yang* via BL 63 and SI 10; and *shao yang* via the gall bladder and Triple Energizer points.

Symptoms that can arise from this meridian
They are mainly superficial, e.g. skin conditions such as acne or boils. Also some types of arthritis in which the joints are not hot as when *yang chiao mai* is involved. Pain experienced along the gall bladder channel of the legs and the lateral aspect of the cervical spine.

The key point is TE 5 (*waiguan*). This is the *lo* point of the TE with which there are strong connections.

3.8.8 *Yin wei mai* (Figure 3.22)

This can be considered a secondary vessel of the kidney. As *yang wei mai* controls the superficial *wei qi* so *yin wei mai* controls the deeper *yin* energy in the meridians.

Course
It starts at KI 9 (*zhubin*) and ascends to the abdomen to SP 13 (*fushe*), SP 15 (*daheng*), SP 16 (*fuai*) and LR 14 (*qimen*), thence to CV 22 (*tiantu*) and CV 23 (*lianquan*).

Symptoms that can arise from this meridian

- Pain in the area of the heart.
- Heaviness in the chest with difficulty in respiration.
- Aching around the waist.
- Pain in the genitalia.
- Diarrhoea, rectal prolapse.
- Thyroid problems which can be affected through CV 22 and CV 23 (local points).
- Mental depression with other emotions such as fear and apprehension. It has links with the spleen, liver and *ren mai* meridians.

Its key point is PC 6 (*neiguan*). This vessel flows in the *tsui yin* which flows upwards from LR 1 (*dadun*) to PC 9 (*zhongchong*) where it meets the opposing *yang* energy of *chao yang*, which is where the key point lies, PC 6 (*neiguan*) the *lo* point of the PC meridian.

3.8.9 Groupings of the eight meridians

The eight meridians can be grouped in the following ways.

1. *Du mai, ren mai* and *chong mai*, all flow directly from the kidneys into the perineum, ascending the abdomen and spinal column, and are used in clinical practice to treat energy at a deep level.
2. *Yin chiao mai* and *yang chiao mai* are complementary to each other, flowing up either side of the legs and ascending to the eyes. In conditions such as insomnia, the possibility of too

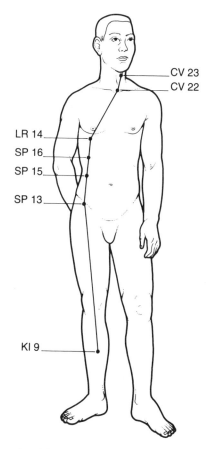

Figure 3.22 *Yin wei mai* (*yin* regulating vessel).

much energy in *yang chiao mai* or in sleepiness and excess in *yin chaio mai* should be considered.

3. *Yin wei mai* and *yang wei mai* complement each other in that they link the *yin* and *yang* meridians respectively.
4. *Dai mai* is a vessel on its own as it girdles the body and connects both *yang* and *yin* meridians as they pass up and down the abdomen. It is of importance in the circulation in the legs.

The eight extra meridians can also be paired according to polarity, i.e. both *yin* or both *yang* as below:

> (a) Du mai *paired with* yang chiao mai. *SI 3* (houxi)/*BL62* (shenmai).

Affecting: posterior aspect of the legs, spinal column, head, eyes and brain.

This pair are particularly indicated in generalized joint disease, e.g. rheumatoid arthritis. The command points of both meridians are treated and points relevant to particular areas added. In the lower limb BL 61 (*pushen*), BI 59 (*fuyang*) and the upper limb SI 10 (*naoshu*), LI 15 (*jianyu*), LI 16 (*jugu*).

If upper motor neurone disease is present and there is muscle spasm, GV 12 (*shenzhu*) is indicated to affect the spinal cord and GV 20 (*bahui*) to affect the brain.

In clinical practice, treatment can precede a mobilizing and exercise programme planned for the individual patient's needs.

In the case of rheumatoid arthritis results following acupuncture are not so good if the patient is taking steroids. This need not prevent the use of acupuncture but expectation of a speedy improvement needs to be treated with caution.

One of the major aims of treatment in rheumatoid arthritis will be to enable the patient to reduce the amount of pain killing drugs and steroids while enabling a rehabilitation programme to be carried out. In the long term steroids cause osteoporosis and analgesics cause digestive problems. It is accepted in Western medicine that such patients will have to take some sort of anti-inflammatory drug most of the time. Acupuncture while not effecting a cure can enable the patient to cope with less of these potentially damaging drugs but it needs to be carried on throughout the course of the disease. It may be necessary only to see the patient three of four times a year. This should be acceptable to the medical practitioner and patient if reduced drug intake can be maintained.

(b) Ren mai *paired with* yin chiao mai *LU 7* (lieque)/*KI 6* (zhaohai).

Affecting: the abdomen, chest, lungs, throat and face.

Indications: this pairing is most influential on female problems, including menopause, premenstrual tension and fluid metabolism. A classic treatment for fluid retention is moxa to the command points, i.e. LU 7 and KI 6. CV 9 is added, as it is influential on fluid balance in the body.

(c) Dai mai *paired with* yang wei mai *GB 41* (Foot linqi)/*TE 5* (waiguan).

Affecting: outer aspect of leg, sides of body, shoulders and side of neck.

Indications: this pair is important in the treatment of migraines associated with menstrual problems. The combination of the cranial gall bladder points of *yang wei mai* and the control of *dai mai* over the genital area enables this pairing to be potentially very effective in these cases.

(d) Chong mai *paired with* yin wei mai *SP 4* (gongsun)/*PC 6* (neiguan).

Affecting: inner aspect of leg, abdomen, chest, heart, stomach.

Indications: this pair is used when there is a profound lack of *yin* energy in the body. The connection of *chong mai* to the kidneys is important in the circulation of *yuan qi* while the *yin wei mai* through CV 22 communicates with the nervous system.

3.8.10 How the key points are used

Traditionally the 'opening or key' points are used differently according to the sex of the patient. The first key point of the 'pair' to be treated is needled on the left side for men and the paired meridian point on the right. For example, if treating *du mai/yang chiao mai* in a man, the first needle inserted will be into SI 3 (*houxi*) on the left hand and then into BL 62 (*shenmai*) on the outer aspect of the ankle. If treating a women the right hand needle will be inserted first.

3.8.11 Conclusion

In clinical practice it is not usual to use the eight extra meridians in a first treatment. Careful assessment is important initially and then the more profound treatment using these paired meridians can be started. Disturbances of a long term nature are best treated with the eight extra meridians rather than acute short term problems.

REFERENCES

Low, R. (1983) *The Secondary Vessels of Acupuncture*. Thorsons Publishers Ltd, Wellingborough, Northamptonshire.
Maciocia, G. (1989) The eight extraordinary vessels: *J.Ch.Med*; No **29**, 3–7.

4

Traditional examination and diagnosis

There are five golden rules in traditional examination.

1. Look
2. Listen
3. Ask
4. Palpate
5. Pulses

4.1 LOOK

4.1.1 Observation of the general demeanour

As the patient walks through the door one should be looking at gait and posture. Then the colour and quality of the skin and brightness of the eyes should be noted.

What posture, gait, complexion and eyes tell us is detailed below.

(a) Posture

The first sight of any individual can give some clue to the state of qi. For example, rounded shoulders and head poking forward indicate, in musculo-skeletal terms, a postural problem which will lead (if not already) to pain in the neck and shoulders. The joints of the cervical spine will probably show on X-ray the effects of wear and tear.

Looking at posture from the traditional Chinese point of view, the rounded shoulders will indicate a lack of qi in the body which causes the postural muscles to be weak. A possible explanation for the posture could be that the governor meridian which passes up the midline posteriorly and/or the bladder meridian which is situated either side of the spine are not supporting the spine. Both are *yang* meridians. Therefore, an initial assessment could be that there is a loss in *yang qi*.

In contrast to the above scenario, the posture could be rigid, upright, and the shoulder girdle raised. This could indicate a hyper *yang* condition.

(b) Gait

This tells us a great deal. There are specific gaits that are associated with various neurological disorders. But there is also the gait that is indicative of the psychological condition of the patient. For example, if the posture described above is combined with a heavy or even a shuffling gait, there could be an element of depression to be considered. Depression is the internal emotion of Earth and the organs paired in this element are the ST and SP.

The controlling influence across the *ko* cycle is GB and LR. Could the apparent postural muscle weakness be the result of a disturbance in the Wind element under which the muscles and tendons are influenced? In contrast an upright stiff posture with raised shoulder girdle accompanied by a hurried/brisk gait could indicate a tense over-anxious person which could be associated with fear, which is the internal emotion of the Water element, the organs of this element being the BL and KI. There could also be an effect across the controlling *ko* cycle which brings in the Fire element or in the mother/son cycle, which would involve the Metal (mother) or Wood (son).

All this information is available to the observant practitioner before greetings have been exchanged.

(c) Complexion

The observation of the overall colour of the skin combined with the quality of the colour can indicate imbalance in the organs. Knowledge of the Five Element Correspondences is again very important. For example, a dull grey complexion combined with dark shadows under the eyes indicates problems in the Water element whose organs are KI and BL and the associated colour is blue/black.

If this is combined with the sagging posture described above this would indicate a very strong Water influence in the condition. A ruddy complexion with red cheeks indicates a strongly *yang* influence together with some disturbance in the Fire element whose organs are SI, HT, PC, TE. The colour of Fire is red. The high colour also indicates rising *qi*. This type of complexion could well be combined with the brisk, tense posture described above.

A white transparent skin could indicate a disturbance in the Metal element, whose organs are LI and LU and the colour associated with that element is white. A person who suffers with pulmonary tuberculosis has an underlying whiteness of complexion even though it can be accompanied with high colour of the cheeks.

A yellowish or muddy complexion could indicate an Earth problem, the organs being ST and SP and the colour yellow.

A greenish complexion can indicate disturbance in Wood whose organs are LR and GB and the associated colour is green. The most obvious example is that of a patient who has hepatitis who has a yellow/green skin colour.

(d) Eyes

The eyes are the outward expression of the internal health or otherwise of the individual. The influencing organs are the liver and gall bladder which are linked in the Wood element.

If there is a lack of clarity in the cornea and a dullness of expression, there is most likely to be some disturbance in the Wood element. The other meridians which are surrounding the eyes should not be ignored. The GB, BL, ST, TE and GV can all influence the eyes.

4.1.2 Tongue diagnosis

The tongue is a visual expression of the balance of meridian energies. It is divided into specific areas, each associated with a meridian (Figure 4.1).

The shape, size, basic colour and coating all are significant. Another important factor is that short term events do not alter the

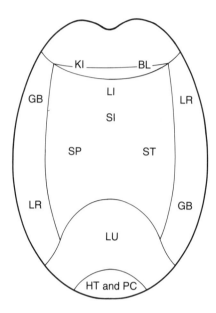

Figure 4.1 Diagnostic areas of the tongue, showing meridians associated with different areas.

tongue. Strenuous exercise for example, will produce a rapid pulse but will not change the shape or colour of the tongue.

The tongue appearance is useful in monitoring the improvement or decline of the patient's condition, the colour of the tongue indicating the chronic condition, the coating being generally more useful in gauging acute conditions.

Examination of the tongue

It is important that there be good lighting and that the tongue is extended for only a short time otherwise the appearance will become more red, especially at the tip, and thus distort the diagnosis.

Differentiating the subtle differences in tongue colour needs a great deal of practice but once mastered can prove a very useful tool in estimating the true energy balance of the organs. NB Medicines can affect the appearance of the tongue causing peeling or thickening of the coating.

There are five important aspects to look for in tongue examination:

1. the vital colour;
2. the colour of the body;
3. the shape;
4. the colour of the coating;
5. the surface moisture.

1. The vital colour
In a condition of disease a good prognosis can be expected if the colour of the root of the tongue is a lively red colour. If there is a withered dark red and dry look the prognosis is poor.

2. The colour of the body
This reflects the condition of the *yin* organs. It is a good guide to the state of the body as it is unaffected by secondary and short term factors. The colours can be described as pale, red, dark red, purple and blue.

The pale tongue: This is indicative of deficiency of blood and *yang qi*. If pale and wet this indicates an inability of spleen *yang* to transform and transport fluids allowing them to accumulate on the tongue. A clinical manifestation could be lassitude, lack of appetite and coldness in the limbs.

The pale dry tongue usually indicates blood deficiency. Blood and fluids are so closely related that one can often lead to another.

The red tongue: Indicates the presence of heat. This will be excess heat if there is a coating. If there is heat from deficiency of *yin* there will be no coating.

Red points or spots indicate blood stasis.

The purple body: Indicates blood stasis which could be from internal cold if it is bluish purple, or from heat if it is reddish purple. The blue body indicates blood stasis from internal cold.

3. The shape
The body shape reflects the state of the organs, *qi* and blood. It is particularly useful in differentiating between excess and deficiency.

A normal tongue should be soft and supple without being flabby, the surface unbroken by cracks. From the eight principles of diagnosis, the clinical significance of the tongue body is that it reflects deficiency or excess in the body. In addition it reflects the state of the organs, *qi* and especially the blood.

The thin tongue: If thinner than is considered normal this indicates a deficiency of *yin* in either blood or fluids. This is explained by the fact that the size of the tongue is determined by the normal supply of blood and fluids.

The swollen tongue: If swollen it means that too much fluid reaches it. This can occur for two different reasons. Either *yang qi* is deficient and fails to transform and transport the fluids which accumulate in the tongue, or there is heat in the body which pushes the heat up to the tongue. A partially swollen tongue can be an important guide to diagnosis. If the edges are affected this indicates a deficiency of spleen *qi* or spleen *yang*.

The area of the partial swelling can be related to the organ which is represented by that area.

The stiff tongue: If the tongue is stiff it always indicates a disharmony of the internal organs. It arises either by excess of heat (when the tongue is red in colour), or internal Wind (indicated by a tongue of pale or normal colour). General signs of heat injuring body fluids could be stiffness in the muscles and difficulty in walking. Signs of the Wind invasion include cerebrovascular accident and asymmetric facial paralysis.

The flaccid tongue: A flaccid tongue should not be confused with a normal tongue in that it lacks normal mobility.

A pale flaccid tongue indicates heart and spleen debility, both these organs being primarily concerned with the blood. The resulting signs and symptoms could be general weakness and in more severe cases muscle atrophy. Other manifestations could include insomnia, lassitude and loss of appetite, and it is also combined with a weak pulse.

A red and flaccid tongue indicates an excess of heat in the tissues. The resulting signs could be similar to those described for the pale tongue but also there may be an impairment to walking.

The long tongue: It is so described when the root is clearly visible on protrusion. It is usually indicative of a hot condition. Clinical manifestations include insomnia, dryness of the mouth, thirst and mouth ulcers.

The short tongue: This can be described as one that cannot be fully extended. It is indicative of both a deficiency and an excess condition. It can be short because there is not enough suppleness due to the body fluids being exhausted by excess heat. It can also be affected by internal cold which has the effect of stiffening the muscle and sinuses, thus restricting its extensibility.

A short pale tongue indicates a deficiency of *qi* and *yang*. It is usually related to deficiency of spleen or kidney *yang*.

If the tongue is red and short, it is the result of internal heat which by disturbing the liver gives rise to internal Wind. This type of tongue is common following a Windstroke or, in our terms, a cerebrovascular accident.

A swollen short tongue indicates a deficiency of spleen or lung *yang* which fails to transform the fluids and forms damp phlegm. This reduces the extensibility of the muscles and tendons.

4. The coating
The tongue coating is produced by the activity of the stomach as a result of its digestive function. If it is white, this indicates a cold condition; if it is yellow, this is indicative of a hot condition.

An analysis of the coating of the tongue indicates the state of the *yang* organs rather than the *yin* organs, which are better assessed through the body colour.

As a general rule the coating is of significance in acute conditions whereas the tongue body colour is of significance in chronic conditions.

White coating: A thin white coating is normal. If thicker it can indicate a cold condition probably affecting the lung or large intestine, white being the corresponding colour of the Metal element. In terms of clinical practice a patient attending for treatment with a feeling of debility and coldness and showing a thickened white tongue coating on a normal colour tongue will probably be suffering from a cold virus. However if the basic tongue colour is pale then this could indicate a more profound condition involving the blood.

The yellow coating: This indicates a hot condition. It also can be generally interpreted to mean that the disease is interior. The third significant factor is that the colour is that of the Earth element and therefore indicative of spleen or stomach abnormality.

The grey coating: This is indicative of a long-standing condition. A grey dry coating indicates heat and a grey wet coating indicates cold.

The black coating: This has similar indications to that of the grey coating.

All the above colours can be found in combination on the surface of the tongue. The area of the coating can also be significant, each area representing an association with the *zang fu* organs.

Clinically it denotes the health of the *yang* organs (Figure 4.1). It can change quickly unlike the body tongue colour. Thus the immediate results of treatment can be seen in the changing character of the coating. Absence of coating depicts a deficiency, whereas a thick coating indicates an excess. The significance of the coating is important in assessing acute conditions but is of less importance in long-standing chronic syndromes.

5. The surface moisture
This provides an indication of the state of body fluids. A dry tongue indicates a deficiency of fluids while a wet tongue indicates an accumulation of fluids. In terms of the Eight Principles it indicates the relative state of *yin/yang* and hot/cold.

4.1.3 The cracked tongue

This is commonly encountered in clinical practice. The significance of the cracks depends on the underlying colour of the tongue body, the location on the surface and the depth. In general terms, the fewer the number of cracks the less severe the disease.

Long horizontal cracks on a red tongue indicate *yin* deficiency stemming from the kidneys. If the tongue is normal the deficiency stems from the stomach and/or lungs.

Short horizontal cracks indicate similar internal conditions as long cracks. They are usually found on a red tongue and can indicate *yin* deficiency.

Cracks resembling ice floes are frequently found in the elderly and indicate deficiency arising from old age. This type of tongue can also be found in women going through the menopause if the tongue body is red without coating. This indicates an advanced state of *yin* deficiency and gives rise to night sweats and joint pain stemming from exhauston of the *yin* fluids.

Transverse cracks on the side of the tongue indicate a long-standing condition of spleen *qi* deficiency.

The significance of the central crack which is seen on many tongues is dependent on other correlating factors in examination. If combined with a red tongue and an even redder tip it is indicative of heart Fire. This is often caused by deep emotional problems. If seen on a red tongue without coating it indicates a deficiency of kidney *yin* which fails to control heart Fire. This can also result from a long-standing emotional problem and extended periods of overwork.

4.1.4 Summary

(a) The normal tongue

This should have a vital colour especially at the root of the body, indicating adequate supply of heart blood. It should be supple and be free of surface cracks and should be steady when extended from the mouth. The normal coating is thin and white indicating normal digestion is taking place. It should be slightly moist.

(b) Abnormal moisture

The moisture and stickiness of the coating signifies the presence of phlegm or dampness.

(c) The toothmarked tongue (Figure 4.2)

This indicates lack of *qi* and inefficient fluid control allowing the tongue to retain fluid, thus impinging on the teeth. The organs to look at in this case are the SP and KI. This is quite a common finding especially in the middle of the winter when body energies can become exhausted. It is often a finding when a patient presents with a chronic joint problem giving rise to pain.

4.2 LISTEN

In clinical practice, the skill of being able to listen is of vital importance. Chinese traditional diagnosis takes into account not only what the patient tells you, but the manner and tone of voice. Each of the Five Elements have their own type of voice (Figure 4.3). A loud/shouting quality is associated with Wood (GB and LR), a musical quality with Earth (SP and ST), a monotonous tone with Metal (LU and LI), a groaning/whining with Water (BL and KI) and a hearty/laughing quality with Fire (TE, PC, SI, HT).

4.3 ASK

4.3.1 Western diagnosis

There is much that needs to be included under this heading. In Western diagnosis the questions posed are designed to ascertain the nature of the disease, the length of time symptoms have been experienced and the severity of the symptoms. The nature of the drugs taken needs to be known as well as the results of other investigations which may have been carried out, e.g. blood tests, X-rays, allergy testing. Examination of the musculo-skeletal system, to ascertain the state of muscle tone and range of movement in the joints, should also be included.

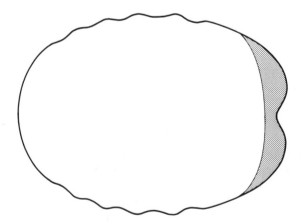

Figure 4.2 A toothmarked tongue.

Influences of Heaven ↓	EARTH	METAL	WATER	WOOD	FIRE	EARTH	METAL	WATER	WOOD	FIRE	←Influences of Earth	
					60-YEAR CYCLE							
FIRE	1924 1984		1936 1996		1948 2008		1960 2020		1972 2032		RAT	HT KI
EARTH		1925 1985		1937 1997		1949 2009		1961 2021		1973 2033	BULL	LU SP
Imperial FIRE	1914 1974		1926 1986		1938 1998		1950 2010		1962 2022		TIGER	TE GB
METAL		1915 1975		1927 1987		1939 1999		1951 2011		1963 2023	HARE	LI ST
WATER	1904 1964		1916 1976		1928 1988		1940 2000		1952 2012		DRAGON	SI BL
WOOD		1905 1965		1917 1977		1929 1989		1941 2001		1953 2013	SNAKE	PC LR
FIRE	1894 1954		1906 1966		1918 1978		1930 1990		1942 2002		HORSE	HT KI
EARTH		1895 1955		1907 1967		1919 1979		1931 1991		1943 2003	SHEEP	LU SP
Imperial FIRE	1884 1944		1896 1956		1908 1968		1920 1980		1932 1992		MONKEY	TE GB
METAL		1885 1945		1897 1957		1909 1969		1921 1981		1933 1993	HEN	LI ST
WATER	1874 1934		1886 1946		1898 1958		1910 1970		1922 1982		DOG	SI BL
WOOD		1875 1935		1887 1947		1899 1959		1911 1971		1923 1983	PIG	PC LR
												DOMINATING ORGANS

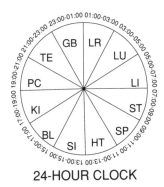

24-HOUR CLOCK

Figure 4.3 The 60-year cycle and 24-hour clock.

4.3.2 Chinese diagnosis

In Chinese diagnosis the questions are initially directed to finding out the individual characteristics of the complaint in relation to the patient's energic make-up. For example, someone born at 1.00 am in April would have a strong Wind bias as this is liver time on the 24-hour clock and springtime according to the month of the year. Even the actual year of birth is important, as each year is influenced by the Five Elements in turn. This is worked out on the 60-year cycle (Figure 4.3).

In this questioning also, the awareness of the influence of the circulation of *qi* through the 24-hour clock (Figure 4.3) and the predominant organs in different seasons of the year is very important. For example, time of day: someone presenting with headaches which are severe in the middle of the day could indicate a disturbance in the GB because at that time *qi* energy is at its minimum in the GB meridian. The path of this meridian is also of significance. The site of the headache then becomes an important aspect of diagnosis. A combination of the time of day described above and a one-sided pain would confirm the impression of a GB problem. The possible cause of the headache could be that insufficient *qi* is reaching the GB between 23.00 and 1.00 hrs and the pain is the result of an empty or *xu* condition. If, however, the pain is felt centrally over the head and the midpoint of the occiput, the governor or bladder meridian could be the meridian which needs attention.

4.3.3 The Eight Principles of diagnosis

The nature of the symptoms needs to be ascertained. For example, if the problem is pain, is it aching/empty or sharp/full? This knowledge will add to the evidence and help to establish a diagnosis based on the Eight Principles, i.e. superficial/deep, *yin/yang*, hot/cold, full/empty. These are described in Chapter 2.

4.3.4 The Six *Chiaos*

Careful questioning to establish the first noticed manifestation of symptoms and subsequent development of signs will help to establish how far the perverse energy causing the signs and symptoms has penetrated. This is described in Chapter 2 dealing with the Six *Chiaos*.

4.3.5 General questions

Under this heading questions as to the general health of the patient are indicated. In a woman the history should include information on her menstrual cycle, obstetric records, etc. These questions are relevant in Chinese diagnosis because it gives a whole picture of the patient and treatment is concerned with the energies in the body as a whole. Questions as to the function of the bowels and bladder are also essential in establishing a diagnosis. The nature of body secretions can add to the overall picture of the patient's health.

When presented with a problem by a patient, in Western practice the inquiry as to the nature of the complaint is confined to the presenting symptoms. In a traditional Chinese history-taking, the function of the whole body energically is of paramount importance. What would appear to be unconnected symptoms can be the clue to the severity or otherwise of body energy imbalance, whereas these same symptoms would be tackled each in its individual way by a practitioner of Western medicine. For example, a patient presenting with pain in the left knee and the right hip, both showing signs of osteoarthrosis, would be treated with local pain relieving treatment and exercises to strengthen the muscles controlling the two joints. Leg length would be assessed and walking re-education, etc. given.

Looked at in the traditional way the Five Element Correspondences are used. Joints are associated with Water and the organs are bladder and kidney. Therefore an assessment of kidney *qi* (the *yin* organ) is indicated. This is achieved through the general questioning combined with tongue and pulse diagnosis. The tongue may well be pale in colour with tooth marks around the edge indicating a *xu* condition. The pulse will feel deep (i.e. that greater pressure is needed to feel the superficial and deep pulses) and the KI and BL pulse particularly weak.

It can be seen that there is a great deal more to ask about in establishing an overall picture of the patient's complaint when embarking on a traditional Chinese diagnosis than in a simple Western style case history. In clinical practice a combination of these two systems can enable the practitioner to treat the underlying energic cause of the problem areas as well as giving practical advice on posture, etc. and treatment to the specific joints.

Under the heading of general questions the diet and lifestyle of the patient should also be ascertained, as this all has a bearing on the problem that is presented.

4.4 PALPATE

4.4.1 Musculo-skeletal

This is carried out to ascertain what tissues are affected. The tension/spasm of the muscle, the mobility/tenderness of joints and the surface feel of the skin should be assessed and noted.

4.4.2 Deep/superficial

The assessment of the level of tenderness in the tissues helps to confirm whether perverse energy has penetrated to the main meridian or is still superficial. For example, pain felt on deep palpation indicates penetration of perverse energy into the main meridian, whereas pain felt on superficial pressure means that perverse energy has not yet reached the deeper main meridian.

4.4.3 Hot/cold

Temperature of the skin will indicate a 'hot' or 'cold' condition. The patient's desire to stretch is indicative of a hot condition whereas the inclination to 'huddle' would demonstrate a cold condition. The temperature of the skin may be the result of a more profound disturbance in body energies. For example, it should be noted that an extreme *yin* condition could give rise to a fever, and the skin feel hot.

4.4.4 Full/empty

If there is a 'full' condition the patient will not like to be touched, but in an 'empty' condition the patient likes to have the painful area pressed.

4.4.5 *Yang/yin*

In a *yang* condition as in a full condition the patient does not like to be touched. Pressure is welcomed on a painful area in a *yin* condition.

4.4.6 Abdominal diagnosis

There are specific areas on the abdomen associated with the various organs of the body (Figure 4.4). Examination of these areas should ascertain the quality, temperature, colour and tenderness of these areas.

4.4.7 *Mu* points

These are the alarm points of the organs. If found to be tender it indicates a disorder associated with the organ (Figure 4.5).

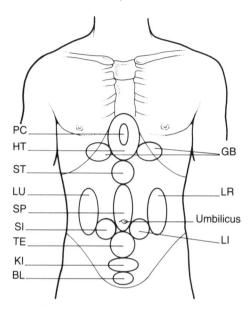

Figure 4.4 Abdominal diagnosis: different areas of the abdomen are considered to be associated with different organs. PC, pericardium; HT, heart; ST, stomach; LU, lung; SP, spleen; LR, liver; SI, small intestine; LI, large intestine; TE, triple energizer; KI, kidney; BL, bladder.

4.4.8 Back *shu* points/associated effect points

These are palpated to elicit the level of sensitivity or tenderness which will indicate a problem with the associated organ. It should be noted that these points in many cases lie directly over the facet joints of the spine and tenderness can be elicited as a result of a facet joint problem. An alternative way to look at this local tenderness is that the therapist is eliciting tenderness in the back *shu* point and involvement of the associated organ. Maitland mobilization on the point could be regarded as acupressure on the back *shu* point or accessory movement of the underlying facet joint. Another bridge between Western and traditional Chinese medicine is the fact that in many cases the sympathetic nerve supply exits at the same levels as the back *shu* points associated with the organs, e.g. BL 13 is at the level of T3 and T4, which is the same as that of the sympathetic nerves which supply the heart and lungs.

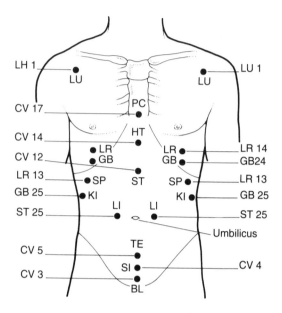

Figure 4.5 *Mu* points and their associated organs. LU, lung; PC, pericardium; LR, liver; GB, gall bladder; ST, stomach; TE, triple energizer; SI, small intestine; BL, bladder.

4.5 THE CHINESE PULSES

This forms an important part of traditional examination, as the quality of the pulses gives a clue as to the nature of the energic disturbance in the body and helps in the assessment of the problem according to the eight approaches to diagnosis.

At each wrist six pulses can be identified reflecting the energy in the twelve organs of the *zang/fu* system (Figure 4.6). Pulses are best felt after the patient has settled down for a few minutes.

4.5.1 Method of taking pulses

The pulses are felt on the brachial artery at the wrist. Three fingertips are placed together over the artery lightly, the three pulses felt under each finger tip at this stage being the *fu* pulses. On the right wrist distal to proximal, they are large intestine, stomach and triple energizer. Similarly, the left superficial pulses are small intestine, gall bladder and bladder.

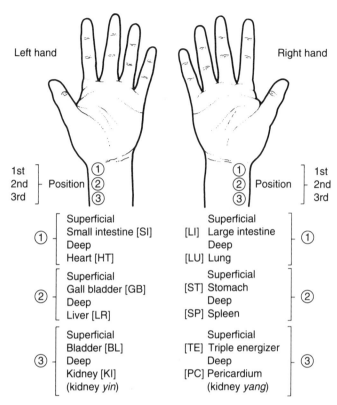

Figure 4.6 The Chinese pulses. Six pulses can be felt at each wrist, associated with different organs.

Each finger tip is then pressed firmly to obscure the pulse and then the pressure is slowly released; the resulting pulse felt is that of the paired *zang* organ. Additionally the level KI *yin* energy is represented by the kidney (deep) pulse on the left and the kidney *yang* energy by the pericardium (deep) pulse on the right wrist.

There is some doubt expressed as to the validity of this diagnostic procedure and there is also a high degree of skill that needs to be developed to feel any difference at all in these pulses and to accurately interpret the findings. However, it is important to know of this examination technique and many practitioners do use this as an essential part of their examination procedure.

4.5.2 *Acabana*

This technique was developed in Japan. It involves finding out how much energy there is in the meridian by heating the *tsing*/nail point.

An **acabana** stick is used. This is rather like a small incense stick, which is lit and then kept glowing. The glowing end is then held over the *tsing* point for a moment and then lifted away. This is repeated until the patient feels hot on that point. This procedure is repeated for all the *tsing* points. (NB the kidney has no *tsing* point but for *acabana* the medial nail point of the little toe is used.)

The number of times needed to heat the point is the energy indicator. If energy is low then more applications are necessary, if high, then less are needed. An imbalance is said to be proved if there is a difference of two in the scores noted for each point.

It should be borne in mind that this method estimates energy in the meridian, whereas pulse taking is finding the energy level in the organ.

4.5.3 What can the taking of pulses reveal?

There are various indicators that can be differentiated when taking the pulses. Invasion of perverse energy can affect the 'feel' in the following way:

Wind – floating pulse;
Cold – slow pulse;
Fire – rapid pulse;
Damp – weak and slippery.

Pulses can also be described in terms of superficial and deep. A superficial pulse can be felt with very little pressure whereas a deep pulse can only be found with a firm pressure of the fingers. In more advanced pulse diagnosis there are even finer distinctions to be felt in both the superficial and deep readings.

It is very useful to be able to feel the different overall quality of the pulses, as this gives a clue to the nature of the invasion of perverse energy. For example, a greasy tongue with a yellow fur combined with a 'slippery' pulse gives a clear indication of damp/heat. In working out a treatment programme therefore acupuncture points specific for affecting this condition can be used.

In classic writings it states that pulses should be felt at dawn. In clinical practice this is clearly not practical. There is also the effect of regular and periodic drugs on the meridian system which can distort the pulse readings.

Many practitioners find that the tongue is a more reliable guide to the relative energy levels in the meridians. Personal clinical experience is, that given the patient is not on regular hormone therapy, e.g. cortisone, HRT, or on a course of antibiotics, it is worthwhile to attempt to take the Chinese pulses in combination with tongue assessment. It is exciting to feel an imbalance and work out how to resolve the problem, then to retake the pulses and to find that they are balanced.

4.5.4 What influences the pulses?

(a) Time of day

If taking pulses it should be noted that the time of day will affect the strength of the individual pulses. Thus between 15.00 and 17.00 hrs one would expect to feel a stronger bladder pulse, according to the 24-hour circulation of *qi* (Figure 3.5).

(b) Time of year

If the patient is coming for treatment in August one would expect the *qi* to be greatest in the organs of the Fire element, i.e. HT, SI, TE and PC according to Five Element theory. If in fact these pulses feel much weaker than the other pulses an imbalance in energy is demonstrated and depending on the symptomology, a treatment plan can be devised.

If the bladder pulse is felt to be weak at a time when it should be strong, e.g. 30th December, and there are symptoms which could arise from lack of *qi* in the Water element pulses, e.g. arthrosis or stress incontinence, adjusting of energy *qi* in the meridian system should be seriously considered.

(c) Drugs

This has been briefly addressed above. If steroids are being taken there is a uniformity in the feel of the pulses and the variables appear to be eliminated. Beta blockers have a similar distorting effect. It is essential to know what drugs have been prescribed.

4.5.5 How can the pulse diagnosis be used in a treatment programme?

Where there is weakness there should be a corresponding fullness in one of the other pulses. Treatment should then be planned to move the *qi* through the meridian system from the stronger to the weaker organ. This manipulation can be achieved in two main ways.

(a) Sheng *cycle*

This uses the concept of Mother and Son. Energy is moved clockwise through the *sheng* cycle. In practice the *sheng* cycle is used to manipulate *qi* in the *yang* (*fu*) organs. Thus the mother of LI is ST and ST is itself son of the TE/SI. For example, a full ST pulse accompanied by a weak LI pulse could mean that there is a stuck energy and to draw it through the mother/son cycle, a point which connects with the mother ST (Earth) and the son LI (Metal) should be used. This is called the tonification point and in this example it is LI 11 (*quchi*).

Each meridian has five command points, one identified with each element. Thus, the Earth point on the LI meridian will draw energy from the ST into the LI.

The command points are listed in Tables 3.1 and 3.2.

(b) Ko *cycle*

This is the controlling cycle in the *zang/fu* system (Figure 2.2), e.g. if the spleen pulse is overfull and the kidney pulse is weak, this could mean that the Earth is suppressing the Water across the *ko* cycle. To restore balance the kidney should be tonified first and the pulses checked. If there is still an imbalance the spleen should be sedated.

4.6 CONCLUSIONS

It can be seen that there is a great deal of information needed before an effective treatment programme can be worked out.

T.C.M. EXAMINATION SUMMARY

Name: _____   Referred By: _____

Address: _____   Western Diagnosis: _____

Occupation: _____   X ray: _____ Date: ____

D.O.B. _____   Time of Birth: _____   Date: _____

SUBJECTIVE

Nature of Complaint: GENERAL HEALTH:

Trauma?

History: PAST HISTORY:

Onset: Sudden, Gradual

Present State: Better, Worse, Static

External Perverse Influences:

  Worse: Heat, Damp, Dry, Cold, Windy.   DRUGS:
  Internal Emotions:
  Happy, Depressed, Grieving, Fearful, Angry/irritated

NATURE OF PAIN   SITES OF PAIN AND
                           PARAESTHESIAE

Sharp, Dull, Constant, Intermittent, Burning

TIME OF DAY WHEN SYMPTOMS ARE MOST SEVERE

```
              24
        23          13
    22  11  12  1   14
        10      2
    21   9       3  15
         8      4
    20    7  6  5   16
        19          17
              18
   Better  Hot  Cold  Pressure
```

Figure 4.7 Examination chart, summarizing the methods of traditional Chinese medicine.

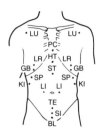

MU POINTS

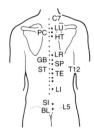

SHU POINTS

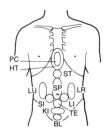

ABDOMINAL AREAS

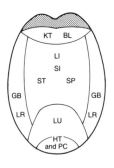

TONGUE:

Shape: long thin swollen toothmarked pointed

Colour: Normal red, pale purple

Coating: Normal, white, yellow on coating,
           greasy, wet dry.

Area of coating: see Diagram

PULSES:

Rapid, slow, deep, superficial, floating
wiry, slippery, full, empty.

	LEFT		RIGHT	
	SI	HT	LU	LI
	GB	LR	SP	ST
	BL	KI	PC	TE
	KI	yin	KI	yang

DIAGNOSIS

AIMS OF TREATMENT:

FURTHER REMARKS:

At first sight the whole examination appears rather pedantic and time consuming. In practice the various observations and questions take little more time than Western style examination. It requires keen observation of the individual while taking a case history and being aware of the extra information that in the light of traditional Chinese diagnosis can be ascertained when examining the patient physically.

All this information needs to be recorded and a suggested examination form is included in this Chapter (Figure 4.7).

5

Technique of treating acupoints with needles and non-invasive procedures

TREATMENT USING NEEDLES

5.1 HYGIENE

The treatment area should be uncluttered so as to avoid dust. The treatment table can be covered with a disposable sheet or have a surface that can be washed after each treatment is finished. Inserting needles into the skin is an invasive procedure and the same careful precautions as would be taken when giving an injection should be observed.

The major problems arising out of invasive techniques are the body fluid borne infections such as hepatitis B and the HIV virus. These can be passed from one individual to another through body fluids. The spore of hepatitis has to be submitted to moist heat in an autoclave before it is destroyed (Table 5.1). The AIDS virus is not so resilient but the same sterilizing procedure is recommended as for hepatitis. The needles themselves have to be carefully cleaned before being autoclaved, as any residue on the shaft could cause tissue damage and discomfort when used again. The most efficient way to clean any residue from the needles prior to autoclaving them is to put the needles in an ultrasound bath.

Many practitioners are now using ready sterilized disposable needles. This greatly simplifies the practice of acupuncture and ensures that there can be no cross infection. **The safest way to practise is to assume that the patient is a carrier of the HIV virus or hepatitis.**

Table 5.1 Use of autoclave

Temperature (°C)	Minimum holding time after temp. achieved (min)
121	15
126	10
134	3

1. Care must be taken by the practitioner to cover any cuts or abrasions on their own hands prior to treating the patient.
2. Discarded needles should be put in a needle safe which is then sealed and incinerated. If blood is drawn a sterile swab should be ready to clean the area. This can then be disposed of in the needle safe.
3. Wash hands thoroughly.

5.2 THE PATIENT

Before embarking on any procedure, the patient must be made fully aware of what is happening and the possible results of treatment.

Contra-indications to treatment with acupuncture needles are

1. first twelve weeks of pregnancy (see Part Three);
2. putting needles into areas of swelling;
3. allergy to stainless steel;
4. piercing infected tissue;
5. needle phobia;
6. there are also acupoints that need to be needled with great care, e.g. those near to arteries and on the thorax.

It is important to note when treating children, that the parent/guardian's written consent to the procedure is recommended. In the United Kingdom it is a legal requirement to obtain such consent.

Symptoms may be exacerbated after a first treatment or there could be some fatigue experienced. It is better to use as few needles as possible initially in case there is a reaction to the acupuncture. It is always safer on a first treatment to lie the patient down. There are some who will react to needles by feeling faint and nauseous and it is easier to deal with these problems when the patient is supine.

There are some patients who are sensitive to stainless steel and in these cases acupuncture would be contra-indicated. Stimulation of the acupoints would have to be attempted using non-invasive methods. It is possible to obtain gold or silver needles which are reusable but this can be very expensive and potentially hazardous, as these needles become brittle after repeated autoclaving and can break in the tissues.

The patient should also be aware of any adverse effects that might occur after treatment. There may be an initial feeling of tiredness and possibly an increase in the presenting symptoms over the following 24 hours. Others may not feel any immediate benefit. All these responses should be made clear to the patient before the end of the first treatment.

5.3 LOCATING THE ACUPOINT

Accuracy is important and the Chinese descriptions of the location of acupoints are very precise. The nearest anatomical surface mark is described and the position of the point from this landmark measured in *cun* (Figure 5.1).

A *cun* is the length of the middle phalanx of the index finger of the patient (Figure 5.2). If an inch measurement were given, this would mean that no account could be taken of the height of the patient. By using the patient's own anatomical measure the acupoints can be accurately located.

While the text books and body charts will give the location of the acupoint, the actual insertion of the needle is governed by the practitioner's own sensitive palpation of the area. A simple light stroke along the line of the meridian should elicit a small area where there is some surface resistance. The finger will appear to stick on the location of the acupoint. Many points are located in natural anatomical depressions in the skin's surface.

Some practitioners use point locators. These are electrical devices which detect areas of reduced electrical resistance on the surface of the skin. Such areas are indicated by a visual indicator or sound. There is some doubt as to the accuracy of these devices and physiotherapists who are skilled in the use of their hands and have a developed sense of touch should not need to use point finders.

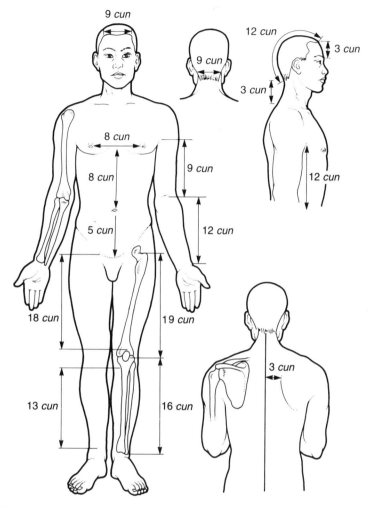

Figure 5.1 *Cun* measurements of various parts of the body.

5.4 ANGLE OF INSERTION

This varies according to the area being treated. The standard texts of TCM describe both the location of acupoints and the angle of insertion (Figure 5.3). There are some practitioners who advocate that the needle should be inserted in the direction of the flow of energy if the purpose is to stimulate the meridian flow, e.g. if needling ST 36 (*zusanli*) which is located 3 *cun* below the knee

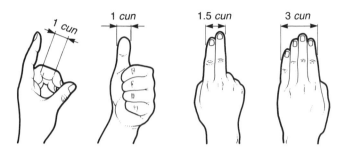

Figure 5.2 Determination of the *cun*, the Chinese unit of measurement, which is determined from the finger size of the individual patient.

between the heads of the tibia and fibula, the direction of the flow of energy in the ST meridian is toward the foot, therefore the needle is inserted in that direction. If a 'reducing' treatment is needed then the direction of insertion would be towards the knee, which is against the flow of energy.

5.5 THE ACUPUNCTURE NEEDLE

Unlike a hypodermic needle the acupuncture needle has a solid shaft. The 'handle' can be of many different patterns. The classic needle has a solid stainless steel shaft with a coiled silver-plated handle which has a loop at the top. The needles are available from approximately 10 mm to 120 mm in length, the diameter from 32 gauge (fine) to 25 gauge (thick). The thickness of the needle is significant in deciding the amount of stimulation required at any

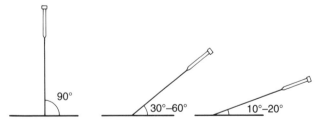

Figure 5.3 The different angles used for insertion of acupuncture needles.

acupoint. It is also easier to handle a thicker needle if a deeper penetration is necessary, e.g. GB 30 lies deep in the gluteus maximus muscle and a needle length of 125 mm is needed. A fine gauge needle would probably buckle when overcoming skin resistance.

The length of the needle chosen should be long enough to locate the acupoint leaving half the shaft exposed. Thus if needling ST 36 (*zusanli*) a 30 mm needle will be necessary as the point lies approximately 15 mm deep in the muscle tissue.

5.6 THE INSERTION OF THE NEEDLE

The needle must be held in such a way as to ensure that the part of the shaft to be inserted into the skin is not touched. Swabbing the skin before insertion of needles is not essential. It has been shown that simple swabbing with an alcohol solution does not sterilize the skin, but local health practice regulations vary and should be studied and conformed to at all times.

Hands must be clean and some practitioners prefer to wear surgical gloves for needle insertion. This is a personal choice. It is difficult to palpate for the acupoint if the fingers are covered but if a point detector is used this need not be a drawback.

In China, it was observed that the experienced acupuncturists carefully located the acupoint and then marked it by holding the handle of the needle and reversing it so that the handle was nearest to the surface of the body. The top of the acupuncture needle was then pressed on to the acupoint. This small depression ensured the accurate penetration of the skin without further feeling for the acupoint.

To prepare for insertion, the handle of the needle should be held between the thumb and index finger of the practitioner's dominant hand (Figure 5.4). The middle finger is placed just below the handle to stabilize the upper third of the shaft. The thumb and index finger of the other hand are placed either side of the acupoint and the skin gently stretched or pinched (Figure 5.5). The point of the needle is then inserted swiftly through the skin. NB The skin on the face usually needs to be pinched prior to needle insertion, whereas the skin on the abdomen, which may be looser, should be stretched.

If the needle is 32 gauge and longer than 30 mm, the tip needs to be supported on the skin's surface, with a sterile cotton wool

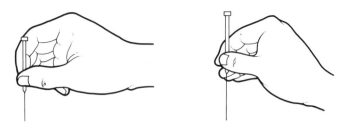

Figure 5.4 The technique used for holding an acupuncture needle.

ball, held between the non-dominant thumb and index finger. An alternative method is to use needles which are ready sterilized with applicator tubes. The tube with the needle inside is then put over the acupoint and the end of the handle tapped to facilitate piercing of the skin. The tube is then removed and the needle inserted to the required depth. Support of the shaft when using longer needles will still be necessary even after using the applicator tubes. The patient sometimes does not feel the entry of the needle but should at any event feel only a small scratching sensation.

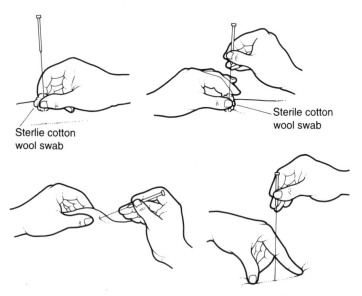

Figure 5.5 Technique for inserting an acupuncture needle.

5.6.1 The plum blossom needle

This is rather like a small double-sided hammer with seven sharp points imbedded on the broad side and a cluster of needles on the other side (Figure 5.6). The acupoint to be treated is lightly tapped to 'supply' and can be 'reduced' by more prolonged tapping to produce a marked erythema.

The original plum blossom needles, which are still available, are made of tortoise shell and have a springy handle, which enables the practitioner to carefully grade the extent of the bounce or percussion over the point. These are not autoclavable and cannot be used in modern safe practice. There can be no objection, however, if the patient keeps their own plum blossom needle and brings it to each treatment. It can be cleaned with 70% alcohol between treatments. Since there is no possibility of anyone else using it there should be no danger of transmitting any blood-borne diseases.

There is available a stainless steel plum blossom needle that is autoclavable; however, it is much heavier to use and treatment more difficult to grade.

5.7 TREATMENT OF THE ACUPOINT

Having pierced the skin the needle is gently thrust down to the required depth and manipulated until the patient feels a dull ache or heaviness around the needle. This sensation is called *'deqi'* and should always be elicited for effective acupuncture treatment. A skilled practitioner can insert the needle to gain *'deqi'* at the acupoint and also achieve a sensation along the line of the meridian. The needle can then be further manipulated to cause an increased sensation of aching or heaviness by rotating the handle slowly for up to two minutes depending on the patient's toler-

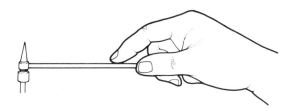

Figure 5.6 The plum blossom needle.

ance, or a similar effect can be obtained by withdrawing and thrusting the needle in the acupoint. These are called reducing techniques. The simple achieving of *deqi* by inserting the needle and leaving it *in situ* without manipulation opens up the meridian pathway. This is described as a 'supplying' technique. When the needle is manipulated the tissues around it appear to tighten and it becomes 'stuck'. After a period of 15 to 20 minutes the tissue around the needle relaxes its hold and the needle can be easily withdrawn. There are some practitioners who simply achieve *deqi* at the point and leave the needle *in situ* for 15 to 20 minutes. They believe that the needle has a balancing effect and if the point needs 'supplying' it will do so and conversely if the point needs sedation this technique will suffice.

There is much argument about what is meant by supplying and reducing techniques. This arises from our inadequate knowledge of the subtleties of the Chinese language and much is misunderstood in translation. Thus the words 'supplying' and 'stimulating' can be used, or conversely 'reducing' and 'sedating'. For example, use of the word 'stimulate' in the English language means to activate. Therefore manipulation of the needle in the point to produce strong *deqi* should mean that the point is being 'supplied' but the opposite is the case, in fact a strong stimulation of an acupoint has a 'reducing' effect in Chinese terms. The description of the effect is on the energy levels in the acupoint/meridian, not on the activity of the needle itself.

5.7.1 Complications of needling

(a) Stuck needle

This may simply be due to muscle spasm and can simply be 'eased out' gently by reassurance to the patient accompanied by massage to the surrounding area. If the needle has been bent on insertion, gentle manipulation combined with withdrawal should solve the problem.

(b) Broken needle

This is more likely when using autoclaved needles, as these become brittle. The point of entry should be marked and the patient taken straight to the nearest casualty department.

(c) Leaving needles in the patient

In a busy clinic, it is always a possibility. A good way to avoid this is to note on the treatment record the points treated as soon as the needles have been inserted, then to count the number of needles removed after the treatment, double checking in the notes that the numbers tally.

(d) Fainting/nausea

Remove the needles immediately and lie that patient horizontal. NB It is a good plan to treat the patient lying down during the first treatment.

5.8 NON-INVASIVE METHODS OF TREATING ACUPOINTS

5.8.1 Moxabustion

Moxa is the name given to the dried material which is derived from the common wild plant *Artemisia vulgaris* (mugwort). It is used as part of acupuncture. It comes in two main forms, moxa punk and moxa rolls.

(a) Moxa punk

The can be used directly on to the skin. A small pyramid shape is formed from the loose fibre and placed on the skin over the acupoint (Figure 5.7a). It is then lit and left *in situ* until the patient indicates that it feels **hot**. It is then removed (quickly) with tweezers. The whole process is repeated a number of times. This number is arrived at by dividing the patient's age by seven if she is a women and by eight if he is a man. Skilled practitioners can treat several points at the same time but it is safer to concentrate on one at a time. There is a real danger of burning the patient if reactions are slow.

There is a second way in which moxa punk can be used. A small amount can be pressed around the top of the acupuncture needle already inserted in the acupoint (Figure 5.7b). This is the reason for having a loop at the top of the handle of the needle – it facilitates the attachment of the moxa to the handle. The moxa is then ignited and allowed to burn out. The needle is heated and

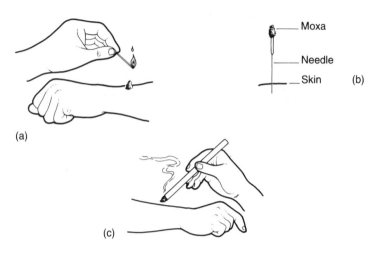

Figure 5.7 Technique for applying moxa; (a) directly onto the skin, (b) via a needle, (c) using a moxa roll.

heat is transmitted directly to the acupoint. Heat is a form of energy and it would only be used when a 'cold' condition is diagnosed.

There is a very useful technique for osteoarthrosis. Points around the affected joint are identified and treated with the needles. The procedure of heating the needles with moxa is carried out three times in 20 minutes. This means that there is an alternate heating and cooling around the acupoint. This seems to have a very beneficial effect on pain and stiffness. The main drawback to this treatment is the danger of hot moxa falling onto the skin during treatment. To prevent this, a shield can be made to protect the surrounding area. A simple solution is to use the thick foil cover of a sterile swab which has a simple cut in one side so that it can be fitted around the needle. Heated needles are an important part of acupuncture and can produce worthwhile results.

(b) Moxa roll

These rolls look rather like large cigars. They are moxa punk which has been moulded into a cylinder shape that can be lit at one end. The moxa roll can now be used to heat acupoints but the glowing end is held about an inch away from the skin (Figure

5.7c). The patient then indicates when the acupoint is hot. The ends of the needles can also be heated by the moxa roll in this way to simulate the more risky technique of burning moxa punk on the end of the needles, described above.

Another useful technique is to cut a small chunk from the moxa roll and wedge it onto the needle handle and light it. This will give a steady heat through the needle for up to 15 minutes and this can be very effective in treating 'cold' conditions such as chronic arthritic joints.

(c) Contra-indications to moxa

1. Loss of skin sensation
It is obvious that to treat any area of the body with moxa that has faulty sensation is foolhardy, especially when the feeling of warmth from the treatment is the practitioner's guide to when to remove the burning moxa.

2. Diabetes
Great care should be taken when using moxa especially on the hands and feet if there is underlying diabetes. Sensation again can be faulty, but the loss of peripheral circulation which is a symptom of diabetes can inhibit the dispersal of the heat from the area and cause a burn which will be difficult to heal.

3. The fumes from burning moxa
Many patients dislike the aroma of moxa. There are now smokeless moxa sticks available on the market which minimize the fumes from the moxa. There are also a variety of other gadgets which are marketed to give the same heat as moxa but without any actual burning of the herb. There is also inconclusive evidence of harmful effects on female practitioners who are in constant contact with moxa, causing some menstrual problems.

4. The balance of *yin* and *yang qi*
The application of moxa by whatever method is a technique of putting energy in the form of heat into the meridian system. It should only be used when dealing with a 'cold' condition. If there is excess of heat or *yang* the application of further heat will widen the discrepancy between *yin* and *yang* and increase the symptoms instead of bringing the energy into balance.

An example of a *yang* condition could be abdominal pain which is accompanied by a clean bright red tongue and a weak rapid pulse. The brightness of the tongue is due to excess of *yang* over *yin*. In other words the *yin qi* is being overcome by the overstrong *yang qi*. Giving a treatment using moxa is going to boost the *yang* energy further and increase the discrepancy. The treatment of choice therefore, would be to use needle stimulation to strengthen the *yin* energy.

(d) Treatment comment

1. Low back pain
In China, it was observed that one of the treatments for low back pain was to heat the acupoints BL 23 (*shenshu*) bilaterally using two moxa rolls. BL 23 is an acupoint 1.5 *cun* lateral to the lower edge of the spinous process of the second lumbar vertebra. The smouldering moxa sticks were held for 20 minutes by the practitioner, giving a constant heat over the area. This acupoint is significant as it is the associated effect (back *shu*) point of the kidney organ. In the theory of the Five Elements, the joints are influenced by the *qi* of the kidney. If there is an existing kidney *xu* condition, then heating BL 23 (*shenshu*) is a direct way to give energy to the kidney through heat. The technique of giving the treatment seemed very similar to simple heat treatment as practised in the West.

In our highly technical and modern practice simple heat treatment is often frowned upon as being only a palliative treatment without valid lasting physiological effects. Following such heat treatment patients usually remark how much better they feel. These subjective effects described by our patients have tended to be dismissed and it is current practice in the West to steer away from such passive treatments. Perhaps in the future when more work has been done to validate the effects of acupuncture on the organs and their associations with body tissues, the use of these 'old-fashioned' methods of using heat in a co-ordinated rehabilitation programme will be vindicated.

2. Asthma
In China it was observed that there were many children with asthma. They were treated with herbal medicine and acupuncture very successfully, but many had come to the big city from the

countryside and after a course of treatment, had to return home. Parents were shown how to cope with potential asthmatic attacks in their children. They were advised to heat the back *shu* point of the lung BL 13 (*feishu*) with moxa and to give acupressure on LU 7 (*lieque*) and CV 17 (*shanzhong*).

5.8.2 Cupping

This is a technique to treat acupoints which involves the use of either a bamboo or glass cup. The size can vary from 1 to 3 inches in diameter. The technique of application requires great care (Figure 5.8).

A lighted taper is held in the cup for a few moments and the cup placed over the skin, centring on the acupoint to be stimulated. The cooling air in the cup contracts and the skin is drawn

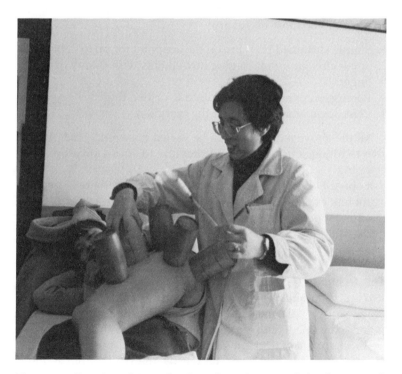

Figure 5.8 Cupping: the cup has been heated using a lighted taper and centred over an acupoint.

up into the resulting vacuum that is created. The length of time that the cup is left depends on the degree of stimulation required.

When removing the cup it should be very gently eased away from the skin while steadying the surrounding tissues with the other hand. The result of this treatment is a strong erythema and sometimes there is also bruising. There is also a danger of causing blisters if the cup is over-heated or left too long *in situ*.

This is a useful technique for large areas such as the lumbar and thoracic spines. It can be used in spinal pain and respiratory disorders, e.g. asthma.

5.8.3 Acupressure

This is a useful technique when it is not possible to use needles. It can be taught to the patient or carer so that they can treat themselves or family at home.

There are various methods of applying acupressure to acupoints. The most useful are:

1. Simple sustained pressure on the acupoint for up to 2 minutes.
2. Small circulatory massaging movements with thumb or index finger.
3. Percussion over the point with one or two fingers.
4. Percussion along the line of the meridian.

All the above techniques can be varied in severity, the percussive techniques from only light pressure to strong pressure as in clapping.

It should always be borne in mind that acupressure is treating acupoints and the same meticulous examination prior to treatment must be made as for invasive acupuncture.

(a) Supplying and reducing the acupoints

The technique of acupressure can be adapted to 'supply' and 'reduce' the points as with acupuncture.

To 'supply' the meridian slow massage is applied over the points combined with prolonged pressure on the skin and, to 'reduce', rapid rotatory movements for only a short time.

The sensation of *deqi* can be felt by the patient, but is more difficult to achieve than with an invasive technique.

(b) *Advantages of acupressure*

1. It is based on the proven efficacy of acupuncture.
2. It is non-invasive.
3. It is a simple skill to learn and to teach lay practitioners, e.g. carers.
4. It can reinforce the effect of acupuncture between visits to the therapist.
5. It can be used when invasive techniques are contraindicated.

(c) *Disadvantages of acupressure*

1. It means a constant presence at the patient's side during treatment which means that only one patient can be treated at a time. With acupuncture, once the needles are inserted, in many cases the patient can be left and another case attended to.
2. Personal experience is that acupressure is not as effective as acupuncture. It is very useful, however, when treating children and anyone who has needle phobia.

(d) *Some particularly useful points which can be effectively treated with acupressure*

The acupoints described below are ones that in clinical practice have been of particular benefit to the patients.

i Nausea

PC 6 (*neiguan*)
Location: 2 *cun* proximal to wrist crease between palmaris longus and flexor carpi radialis.

This point is effective in sickness. In Chinese medicine sickness is due to rising *qi* and over-fullness of the heart. Pressure over PC 6 (*neiguan*) has a calming effect through the pericardium meridian. Examples of conditions which respond to acupressure on this point are:

1. travel sickness;
2. post surgical nausea;
3. nausea experienced in malignant disease;
4. hyperemesis.

A wrist band is now sold commercially which has a small prominence designed to give pressure over this point.

ii Anxiety
HT 7 (*shenmen*)
Location: antero-lateral aspect of the wrist crease, just proximal to the pisiform.

This point is effective for anxiety and insomnia caused by agitation. Massage of this point prior to retiring can assist a good night's sleep. If the point is over-massaged thus 'reducing' the point the effect can be to prevent sleep. For example: a patient in Guanchiao acupuncture clinic was suffering from insomnia among other stressful symptoms. She was given a plum blossom needle to use at home prior to retiring. She was instructed to tap over HT 7 (*shenmen*) 20 times on the right and left wrists. The first night after treatment she slept only fitfully. So the next night she tapped the point many times more and the area was visibly reddened on her next visit to the clinic. She had had no sleep at all and was very tense. The over treating of the point had had the opposite to the desired effect.

iii Pain
LI 4 (*hegu*)
Location: between the thumb and index finger at the crest of the bulge made by the 1st interossius muscle when the thumb is pressed against the index finger (Figure 3.4).

This point has many uses. It is effective in low back pain, headaches, facial pain, and toothache. It is on the LI meridian and can also help in regulating the bowel.

The technique for this point is for the practitioner to locate the point and hold the area between thumb and index finger, squeeze the point and massage it with small circular movements.

iv Neck and shoulder pain
- GB 20 (*fenchi*)
  Location: between the depression directly inferior to the occipital protuberance and the mastoid process and posterior to the transverse process of the atlas vertebra (Figure 3.13).
  This is an important point for muscle spasm of the cervical

region and headaches. The point is easily located and accessible to treat oneself. The techniques described above can all be used with effect. It is particularly effective for the type of headache that is centred on the occiput.

- TE 16 (*tianyou*)
  Location: posterior to the mastoid process and inferior to the origin of the sterno-cleido-mastoid (Figure 3.12).
  This approximates to the apophyseal joint of the 2nd cervical vertebra. In practice this point is inadvertently treated when using Maitland mobilizing procedures. It can produce immediate relief of muscle spasm and increased range of cervical movement. It is also effective for hemispherical headaches. In Western terms rhythmical pressure over this area produces an accessory movement of the apophyseal joint and this has an effect on the surrounding structures, in particular, the 2nd cervical nerve.
  Maitland mobilizations along the cervical thoracic and lumbar spines often coincide anatomically with acupoints. There are many such coincidences to be found in clinical practice.
- GB 21 (*jianjing*)
  Location: at the highest point of the shoulder (Figure 3.13). This is another very useful acupoint which also has a direct relationship with the angle of the first rib. In many years of practising mobilizing/manipulation techniques prior to studying acupuncture, this was found to be extremely useful in releasing muscle spasm in the upper fibres of the trapezius. The interesting question is, does downward pressures over the first rib angle cause a muscle stretching effect thus releasing muscle spasm or does the pressure activate GB 21 and the GB meridian to eliminate an 'invasion of Wind'?

v Respiratory conditions
- CV 17 *shanzhong*
  Located on the sternum at the level of the nipples (Figure 3.16). Acupressure on this point can assist a patient to produce phlegm when the cough is not productive. This is a very useful point as patients can be shown how to stimulate it for themselves.

- BL 13 (*feishu*)
  Location: 1.5 *cun* lateral to the spinous process of T3 (Figure 3.9). Massage of this point can assist during respiratory distress. When treating a post-operative chest infection where effective coughing is painful, massage over BL 13 and CV 17 points can greatly assist the patient to expectorate. These are personel experiences and have not been tested in any clinical trial.
  Heat can also be applied to BL 13 with good effect. Patients suffering with chronic respiratory disease can be shown how to apply this themselves at home using a heat pad or hot water bottle.

Gynaecology
- ST 36 (*zusanli*)
  Location: 3 *cun* below ST 35 and one finger width lateral to the tibial tubercle (Figure 3.5).
  In working with post-operative gynaecological cases there is often a problem with wind and stomach distension. Acupressure on this point will bring almost instant relief in many cases.
- SP4 (*gongsun*)
  Location: medial aspect of foot in a depression at the proximal end of the 1st metatarsal (Figure 3.6).
  This can be effective in lower abdominal pain especially following abdominal surgery.

Pregnancy
The early weeks of pregnancy can be very uncomfortable for some women, who have morning sickness. This is due mainly to weakness of stomach *qi* as a reaction to the fetus. Acupuncture is successful in alleviating these symptoms, but some 'potent' points are not advised for use with needles in the early weeks as they might cause a miscarriage. ST 36 (*zusanli*) and PC 6 (*neiguan*) are two of the major points on which acupressure can be safely applied.

5.9 THE RULES OF ACUPUNCTURE

The rules of acupuncture are for guidance only, when a treatment programme is being formulated.

5.9.1 General rules

(a) Points in area

Local acupoints to the problem area can be used purely for local effect. Several different meridians may be involved. For example, shoulder disorders: LI 15 (*jianyu*), TE 14 (*jianliao*), SI 9 (*jianzhen*), SI 10 (*naoshu*), LU 1 (*zhongfu*). Knee disorders: SP 9 (*yinlinquan*), LR 8 (*ququan*), ST 35 (*dubi*), GB 34 (*yanglinguan*).

(b) Points in line

This method is used when a strong effect is needed on one particular meridian. For example, sciatica: BL 36 (*chengfu*), BL 37 (*yinmen*), BL 40 (*weizhong*), BL 56 (*chengjin*). Lateral leg pain: GB 30 (*huantiao*), GB 31 (*fengshi*), GB 33 (*xiyiangguan*), GB 34 (*yanglinguan*).

(c) End points

These are effective in *yang* conditions. For example, acute eye inflammation: GB 1 (*tongziliao*), BL 1 (*jingming*). Shoulder pain: LU 1 (*zhongfu*).

(d) Local and distal points

There are two established ways of conforming to this rule.

(a) End of meridian points. In this method both end points are needled. For example, hay fever: LI 1 (*shangyang*), LI 20 (*yingxiang*). Headache localized to latter aspect of eye: GB 1 (*tongziliao*), GB 44 (foot *qiaoyin*).
(b) Points in the middle area of meridian. These should be used with the *ho* point. For example, hip pain: GB 30 (*huantiao*), GB 34 (*yanglinguan*) *ho* point. Shoulder pain: LI 11 (*quchi*), LI 15 (*jianyu*).

(e) Points with special action or influential points

These are described in the Chinese texts as having a particular effect on body tissues. For example:

- GB 34 (*yanglinguan*) is the influential point for muscles and tendons.
- BL 40 (*weizhong*) special point for skin disorders.
- CV 17 (*shanzhong*) influential point for respiratory disorders.
- BL 11 (*dashu*) influential point for bone.
- CV 17 (*shanzhong*) influential point for respiratory system.
- BL 17 (*geshu*) influential point for blood.
- GB 39 (*xuanzhong*) influential point for marrow.

(f) Key/confluent points

These are the eight points that are used in activating the eight extra meridians. That is:

- TH 5 (*waiguan*) – *yang wei mai*
- GB 41 (Foot *linqi*) – *dai mai*
- SI 3 (*houxi*) – *du mai*
- BL 62 (*shenmai*) – *yang chiao mai*
- PC 6 (*neiguan*) – *yin wei mai*
- SP 4 (*gongsun*) – *chong mai*
- LU 7 (*lieque*) – *ren mai*
- KI 6 (*zhaohai*) – *yin chiao mai*

(g) Five Element balancing

In this method the *qi* is moved around the *sheng* cycle or across the *ko* cycle by use of the command points of the meridians.

(h) Associated effect points/back Shu points

These are points on the bladder meridian lying 1.5 *cun* lateral to the spinous processes, each with a direct effect on a specific organ.

(i) Formulae

These have been evolved over many years and found to be effective for specific disorders. For example, hay fever: LI 4 (*hegu*), LI 11 (*quchi*), LI 20 (*yingxiang*), *ying tang* (extra point). Anxiety/ tension: LI 4 (*hegu*), LR 3 (*taichong*), GB 34 (*yanglinguan*).

(j) Points on opposite side

It is interesting to note that pain on one side of the body can be successfully treated by needling points on the opposite side. For example, phantom limb pain. This can be effectively relieved by treating local points on the intact limb corresponding to the area of the phantom limb pain.

5.9.2 Forbidden points for needles

1. Any point in an area of swelling, unhealthy skin or varicosities.
2. Nipple and breast tissue. (ST 17 *ruzhong*, the nipple, is forbidden moxa as well.)
3. The umbilicus although moxa on this area can be very effective in *yin* conditions. This is traditionally applied on a piece of root ginger or by filling the umbilicus with salt and putting moxa cones on top.
4. Scalp areas on infants before the fontinelles have closed.
5. The external genitalia.

5.9.3 Vulnerable points

1. Those which enter the eye orbit.
   BL 1 *jingming*
   ST 1 *chenggi*
2. Those in the area of the neck.
   CV 22 *tiantu* (superior mediastinum)
   LI 18 Neck *futu* (over the great vessels of the neck)
   SI 17 *tianrong* (over the carotid body)
   GV 15 *yamen* (over the spinal cord)
   GV 16 *fengfu* (over the brain stem)
3. Those in the area of the chest unprotected by bone or cartilage, e.g. LU 1 *zhongfu*, GB 21 *jianjing*.
4. ST 21 *liangmen* on the right side, as it overlies the *gall bladder*.
5. Points close to blood vessels.
   The blood vessels should be carefully palpated and held clear prior to insertion of needles, e.g. LU 9 *taiyuan*, PC 3 *quze*.
6. LR 3 *taichong*. This can produce over correction of hyperten-

sion, as one action of this point is to reduce blood pressure. It can also cause hypoglycaemia in diabetic patients.

5.9.4 Contraindications to acupuncture therapy

1. **Malignancy**. Acupuncture cannot cure malignancy and any treatment for relieving pain should be given as part of a coordinated treatment programme in close consultation with the medical team.
2. **Pregnancy**. In the first and last three months of pregnancy. Points which are most likely to disturb pregnancy are LI 4 *hegu*, SP 6 *sanyinjiao*, ST 36 *zusanli*, KI 3 *taixi*, KI 6 *zhaohai*, BL 67 *zhiyin*, points of the lower abdomen, ear points related to endocrine and genito-urinary system. Scalp points: genital and foot motor sensory areas.
3. **Drugs**. Practitioners should know what drugs the patient is taking and their effect on the patient. The acupoints can then be chosen to avoid over response to treatment, e.g. in patients on medication for diabetes a hypoglycaemic state may occur.
4. **Haemorrhagic disease**. Invasive methods are best avoided. Laser or acupressure can be used instead.

5.10 CONCLUSIONS

There are several ways in which the principles of TCM can be applied to treatment of patients, using invasive and non-invasive techniques. Careful attention to examination, diagnosis and hygiene prior to commencing treatment is of paramount importance if there is to be a successful outcome.

6

Current practice in China

Since the Revolution in 1949 there has been active encouragement for TCM in China. Government support has enabled research to be undertaken. Much work has been done in the laboratory to validate the effect of acupuncture on pain (Han and Teranius, 1982). There are also a large volume of papers on the therapeutic effects of acupuncture on many medical conditions (O'Connor and Bensky, 1975). However, these are mainly discriptive studies and not in the form of 'trials' using control groups. Other ways of using acupuncture have also been developed, which are not always strictly based on TCM.

6.1 EAR ACUPUNCTURE

This was not developed to any great extent until Nogier's work in France in 1957. Prior to that a brief word in the *Nei Jing* (*The Yellow Emperor's Classic of Chinese Medicine*) and *Zhen Jiu Da Jung* (*Compendium of Acupuncture and Moxabustion*) was the only mention of this now very popular form of treatment. Because there is not a long traditional practice of this particular form of acupuncture, more use is made of Western concepts of medicine when finding and naming points of particular effect in the ear. An example of this would be the endocrine point for menstrual disorders or the sympathetic nerve point for circulatory disorders or muscle spasms. Ear acupuncture will be addressed further in Part Two.

6.2 ANAESTHESIA

Another modern aspect of acupuncture is that of its use in anaesthesia. The pain relieving properties had been well established and accepted and following successful work on post-operative pain the next step was the performing of operations using acupuncture. In 1958 in Shanghai the first operations were performed using acupuncture. In 1983 the author, when studying in Guanchiao, witnessed the removal of a tumour on the thyroid gland. The patient was fully alert and was able to answer questions during the procedure.

The preparation for the procedure using acupuncture involved a minimum of 20 minutes electrical stimulation of needles placed in PC 6 (*neiguan*) and LI 4 (*hegu*) preceded by an injection of Valium. The patient had to lie very still for one hour and a half and was clearly exhausted at the end of the proceedings, but had not been in any pain. It was interesting to note that at that time (1983), most surgical procedures were performed at this particular hospital using conventional general anaesthetic. The early enthusiasm for surgical acupuncture anaesthesia has abated somewhat, although it can be an efficient way to ease pain in some cases.

The author was asked to treat a patient in the UK newly returned from China who had fallen and sustained a Colles' fracture. The accident had taken place in a country area far away from a large General Hospital. The accident happened at 3.00 pm. She was X-rayed at 4.00 pm (a very ancient X-ray machine) and offered acupuncture prior to manipulation of the fracture or a general anaesthetic which could not be administered for a further three hours. She opted for acupuncture. One needle was placed in the supra clavicular fossa (patient's description) and she saw the wrist manipulated and felt the bones move but felt no pain. During the procedure the needle was stimulated manually. She was able to enjoy her supper at 6.30 pm with the post anaesthetic effect of the acupuncture still eradicating the pain. Her recovery on removal of plaster was normal.

6.3 ALTERNATIVE TECHNIQUES

6.3.1 Formula use of acupuncture

Various acupoints have been used in some conditions based on the understanding and practice of TCM. When looking at recommended formulae for various conditions it is sometimes difficult to understand the reason for using the acupoints recommended. It is not possible to practise acupuncture effectively without knowledge of the extra meridian systems which link the main meridians and have a profound effect on the balance of energy in the deeper levels of the body. These extra meridians have been discussed in Chapter 3.

6.3.2 Injecting acupoints

In Guangzhou in 1983 there was much emphasis put on the practice of injecting acupoints. The drugs injected were Chinese herbal remedies which were formulated to enhance the acupuncture for the various conditions treated. There was also frequent use of vitamin B12 to encourage nerve regeneration particularly in facial palsy.

Another radical treatment was that of catgut embedding. This involved injecting sterile catgut into acupoints giving a constant stimulation while the 'irritant' was being absorbed. It was said to be effective for up to 2 weeks after insertion. A simple lumbar puncture needle was used to insert the catgut. There was no local anaesthetic used and the procedure was not a comfortable one for the patient. Extreme care had to be taken when points in the thoracic area were treated.

6.3.3 Laser acupuncture

This is widely used to treat children in China. It is described in Part Two.

6.4 RESEARCHING ACUPUNCTURE

Setting up a study into the practice of acupuncture on human subjects and comparing the efficacy of this treatment with standard Western practice is fraught with difficulty. The discipline of equality for both groups of participating patients means that if a standard Western treatment is used, i.e. medication, then a standard acupuncture treatment should also be used, i.e. using the same points at each visit. The practice of acupuncture is a dynamic procedure and treatment is adapted to the patient's presenting symptoms at each visit. Thus, imposing the same discipline on acupuncture as on Western treatment does not give a fair result. However, the specific effect of some acupoints on some conditions have been researched, with interesting results.

The author became aware of the effect of SP 6 (*sanyinjiao*) in urinary problems over some years of practice. The elderly patients referred for arthritic pain were finding that they no longer had to get up at night to void their bladder, or the number of times this happened during the night was reduced. Treating these patients in the traditional way meant that needles were used local to their painful and distal points to affect the body energies at a deeper level. The acupoint SP 6 (*sanyinjiao*) was used as a point to balance the *yin* and *yang* energy of the kidney. According to the theory of the Five Elements (Chapter 2) the bones and thus the joints are directly influenced by the *qi* of the kidney and the paired bladder organ. It was hypothesized that SP 6 had affected frequency of micturition at night. The efficacy of this point combined with ST 36 (*zusanli*) was tested in a pilot study using a single blind trial design, on elderly residents in long-stay hospitals. ST 36 *zusanli* was added as this is considered a point which if stimulated augments meridian energy. All the acupuncture patients showed reduced incidences of nocturia compared with the control group who showed no change. The results were highly significant but the numbers were very small, 11 in the acupuncture group and nine in the placebo (Mock TENS) group (Ellis, 1993). This is just one example where specific points have been shown to have an effect on body systems and the research was carried out using a standard research protocol.

6.5 SCALP ACUPUNCTURE

The underlying principle behind scalp acupuncture is that specific functional parts of the brain can be affected by stimulating identified areas on the surface of the scalp. In most cases these scalp areas are close to the areas of the brain they represent. This has been a technique of acupuncture which has been developed over the past three decades. The points are located according to the cerebral function areas and have no basis in TCM. Scalp acupuncture is used widely in China for neurological and psychological disorders. There is anecdotal evidence of restoration of speech following cerebrovascular accidents after scalp acupuncture.

There is much research needed in this new field of acupuncture to establish the existence of these functional areas on the scalp and to validate the effectiveness of their inclusion in a rehabilitation programme.

6.6 CONCLUSIONS

Current practice of acupuncture in China is still evolving and new techniques are adopted as research and clinical practice push the frontiers of knowledge further forward.

The TCM hospitals thrive alongside the Western hospitals and Chinese citizens are free to choose where to get advice. Recently (1992) in Nanjing I observed patients in a TCM out-patient clinic being referred for ultrasound examination for investigating gall bladder pain and for ECGs when irregularities were felt in the pulses.

The effectiveness of acupuncture has meant that it has survived through thousands of years. In China today the patient benefits from the combined expertise of traditional and Western trained practitioners.

REFERENCES

Ellis, N. (1993) The effect of acupuncture on nocturnal urinary frequency and incontinence in the elderly. *Complementary Therapies in Medicine*, 1 (3), 168–170.

Han, J. S. and Terenius, L. (1982) Neurochemical basis of Acupuncture analgesia. *Annu. Rev. Pharmacol. Toxicol.*, 22, 193–220.

O'Connor J. and Bensky, D. (1975) A summary of research concerning the effects of acupuncture. *Am. J. Chinese Medicine*, 3(4), 337–394.

Part Two

Concepts of Western Acupuncture

7

Current theories of the physiological effects of acupuncture

Following a period of rejection of acupuncture by orthodox practitioners of medicine, there has been a steady stream of research supporting the fact that there is a significant effect on physiological mechanisms controlling pain when acupoints are stimulated. In the past 17 years there have been many studies in which these questions have been asked:

1. Does acupuncture really relieve pain?
2. How does it work?
3. Do acupoints/meridians really exist?

7.1 DOES ACUPUNCTURE REALLY RELIEVE PAIN?

There is now little doubt that acupuncture can relieve pain by stimulating physiological reactions to an invasive stimulus. Anaesthesia is initiated by stimulation of the small diameter nerves in muscles, which send impulses to the spinal cord. The spinal cord, midbrain and pituitary are then activated to release transmitter chemicals (endorphins and monoamines) which block the noxious impulses.

Nerve fibres are classified by size and according to whether they originate in skin or muscle. Large diameter myelinated nerves A beta (skin) or type I (muscle) carry touch and proprioception respectively. Small diameter myelinated A delta (skin) or types II and III (muscle) carry pain. The smallest unmyelinated C (skin) and type IV (muscle) also carry painful messages. Types II, III, IV and C also carry non-painful messages (Pomerenz, 1990).

7.2 HOW DOES IT WORK?

To get an analgesic effect it is important to achieve *deqi*. This is the dull heavy sensation which is felt around the acupuncture needle when it is moved within the acupoint. If a subcutaneous injection of procaine is given prior to inserting the needle the *deqi* is not affected; however, if a similar injection is given deep into the muscle in the acupoint area there is inhibition of *deqi* (Chiang and Chang, 1973). It can be logically concluded in the light of the above findings that the main components for *deqi* are carried by types II and III afferents (small myelinated afferents from muscle). In the case of those acupoints not sited in muscle the response is through the peripheral nerves so that the A delta fibres are stimulated. Impulses are sent to the spinal cord and at cell 5 the impulses are transmitted up the anterolateral tract to activate three centres:

1. Spinal cord at the lateral horn where enkephalin and dymorphin block incoming messages at low frequency and other transmitters, not fully identified, at high frequency. The analgesic effect of high frequency stimulation is short lived, lasting very little time after the stimulation stops.
2. Midbrain. This uses enkephalin to activate the raphe descending system, which inhibits spinal cord pain transmission by a synergistic effect of the monoamines, serotonin and norepinephrine.

   It also has a circuit which bypasses the endorphinergic links when there is high frequency stimulation.
3. Pituitary/Hypothalamus. The pituitary is where β-endorphin is released into the blood circulation and cerebrospinal fluid, thus completing the pain relieving process from a distance. The hypothalamus has connections with the midbrain and sends out long axons which, via β-endorphin, activate the descending analgesia system. The third centre is only activated at low frequency. The effect of stimulating at low frequency produces a slower analgesic effect which lasts beyond the treatment time. It is cumulative, so the effect is increased with successive treatments.

The significance of identification of three areas enables the analgesic effects of acupuncture to be analysed from a local and distal aspect. Local needling on or near the site of pain works through the lateral horn of the spinal cord primarily and then the midbrain and hypothalamus/pituitary is involved, whereas needling distal to the painful area activates the midbrain and hypothalamus/pituitary. This analgesia will affect the body as a whole.

Analgesia can thus be reinforced by treating both the local and distal area. Western research has demonstrated that Naxalone when introduced into the body inhibits the analgesic effect of acupuncture. This leads to the conclusion that acupuncture stimulates the production of endorphins to produce analgesia, as Naxalone and similar chemical substances are known to block endorphins.

It has also been shown that the release of monoamines (serotonin and norepinephrine) which are produced in the midbrain are increased following acupuncture (Han *et al.*, 1979).

The frequency of electrical stimulation on the surface of the skin also affects different parts of the pain system described above and this will be discussed in Chapter 8.

7.3 DO ACUPOINTS/MERIDIANS REALLY EXIST?

There has been much research into the particular nature of acupoints and experiments comparing the anaesthetic effect of non-acupoint acupuncture with insertion of needles into identified acupoints. In acute pain induced in the laboratory there has been clearly demonstrated a significant analgesic effect with true acupoint acupuncture whereas there has been little effect following 'sham' acupuncture (only 3% of cases) (Chapman *et al.*, 1977).

The results are not so clear, however, when dealing with chronic pain. Here various studies have shown a 33–50% placebo effect in humans. Another important aspect of research has been into the nature of the acupoint. How is it identified and is there a significant anatomical reason for the location of such points?

Researchers led by Professor Zhu Zong Xiang from Beijing took blocks of skin from seven amputated limbs and checked the thickness of the layers of cells in the skin, under a microscope. In 87.4% of an unstated number of samples examined, the skin was thinner along the lines of the meridians as described in traditional Chinese medicine (McKinley, 1991).

On the other hand, a notable experiment in France by Simon and colleagues was to inject the radioactive tracer technetium-99 into an acupoint and trace its path from the area. The same treatment was carried out on a non-acupoint. There was no identified pathway noted in either case other than that through the venous and lymphatic systems (Simon *et al.*, cited by Bensoussan, 1991).

Work is continuing both in China and the West to try to prove the existence of the meridians.

It is interesting to note that in traditional Chinese medicine, when treating pain, one of the basic rules of acupuncture is to use local and distal acupoints. The reasons given are that the pain is present because the energy or *qi* is stuck and cannot flow freely through the meridian. Tapping into the meridian at the local point near to the pain and a distal point along the same channel will facilitate the return to normal energy flow. This copies the Western approach of inducing short-term and long-term analgesia by stimulating the spinal and midbrain reflex to pain respectively.

The important thing is that the treatment is invariably effective whatever the explanation given.

7.4 OTHER POSSIBLE EFFECTS OF ACUPUNCTURE

One should not ignore the possible effect of puncturing the skin producing electrical stimuli which could have a biological effect on nerve regeneration. Nerves grown in cell cultures have been shown to grow towards the negative pole of a weak DC electrical field (Patel and Poo, 1982). The insertion of a needle through the skin causing a small lesion therefore may be causing a negative charge and thus stimulating nerve growth.

There is anecdotal evidence of 100 000 patients in China with Bell's palsy of the 7th cranial nerve benefiting from acupuncture without any electrical stimulation. In Guanciao in 1983 I was treating many such patients who had had long-standing Bell's palsy.

7.5 CONCLUSIONS

Much research has been done using animal studies to identify the mechanisms which have been affected by acupuncture. It has been demonstrated that acupuncture analgesia activates the body's pain modulatory system, thus suppressing the transmission and perception of noxious information at various levels of the central nervous system (Han, 1986).

More research is needed to establish a synthesis of the Western concepts of the effect of acupuncture and the TCM experience. 'It

is comparatively difficult for us to describe the true mechanism of
acupuncture before the theories of the channels are identified by
modern science' (Chen Peixi, 1983).

The emphasis of scientific investigation has shown that acupuncture has an effect on the pain systems of the body, but there
has been little work in the literature of the West referring to the
effects of acupuncture on other disorders, e.g. gynaecological,
respiratory, digestive, immunological, hormonal and allergic
problems. Until there has been satisfactory and consistent proof
produced of the effects of acupuncture on these disorders, the
mainstream of practice will be in analgesia and an important tool
to address non-painful conditions will continue to be neglected in
Western medicine.

REFERENCES

Bensoussan, A. (1991) The nature of the meridian, *The Vital Meridian*,
Churchill Livingstone, Melbourne, Edinburgh, London and New York.
Chiang, C.Y. and Chang, C.T. (1973) Peripheral afferent pathway for
acupuncture analgesia. *Scientica Sinica*, **16**(1), 210–217.
Chapman, C.R., Chen, A.C., and Bonica, J.J. (1977) Effects of
intrasegmental electrical acupuncture on dental pain: evaluation by
threshold estimation and sensory decision theory. *Pain*, **3**(3), 213–227.
Chen Peixi (1983) An Examination of the Differences between Western
Medicine and Traditional Chinese Medicine. Lecture delivered at the
Zhongshan Medical College, Guangzhou, China.
Han, C.S., Chou, P.H., Lu, L.H., LU, C.C., Yang, T.H., and Jen, M.F. (1979)
The role of central 5-HT in acupuncture analgesia. *Scientica Sinica*,
22(1), 91–104.
Han, C.S. (1986) 'Physiological and neurochemical basis of acupuncture
analgesia', in *The International Textbook of Cardiology*, (ed. T.O. Cheng),
Pergamon Press, New York, pp. 1124–1132.
McKinley, P. (1991) Secrets of the life force. *Here's Health*, Jan., 10–11.
Patel, N. and Poo, M.M. (1982) Orientation of neurite growth by
extracellular electrical fields. *J. Neurosci.*, **2**(4), 483–496.
Pomerenz, B. (1990) Scientific basis of acupuncture, in *Basics of Acupunc-
ture*, second revised and enlarged edition, Springer-Verlag, Berlin,
Heidelberg, New York, London, Paris, Tokyo, Hong Kong, Barcelona.

FURTHER READING

Bensoussan, A. (1991) *The Vital Meridian*, Churchill Livingstone, Melbourne, London, Edinburgh and New York.
Stux, G. and Pomerenz, B. (1991) *Basics of Acupuncture*, second revised
and enlarged edition, Springer Verlag, Berlin, Heidelberg, New York,
London, Paris, Tokyo, Barcelona.

8

Electro-acupuncture

8.1 INTRODUCTION

Stimulation of the acupuncture needle by electricity is a modern innovation of acupuncture. It was initially used to simulate a constant manual manipulation of the needle when anaesthesia was desired. The practice of electrical stimulation has grown and developed over the years and now many practitioners use this routinely to supplement the action of the needles. Areas of electrical conductivity are shown in Figure 8.1.

The other important outcome of this technique is that it has enabled carefully controlled experiments to be undertaken in which the specific effects of electro-stimulation on the endogenous opioid peptidergic system can be studied (He, 1987).

There are four ways in which electro-stimulation can be used in clinical practice.

1. To locate acupoints by finding areas of reduced electrical potential on the skin's surface.
2. To stimulate the pain coping mechanisms of the body.
3. To supply or sedate the acupoints.
4. Electro-acupuncture according to Voll (EAP).

8.2 TO LOCATE ACUPOINTS

Simple point finders can be purchased, which either light up or give an auditory indication when the area of skin touched shows a reduced electrical potential from the surrounding tissue, thus indicating an acupoint.

There are other point finders which involve the patient holding an electrode in one hand while the operator moves a probe over the area where the acupoint is located and when the area of decreased electical potential over the acupoint is touched there is an auditory or visual indication by the machine. These machines

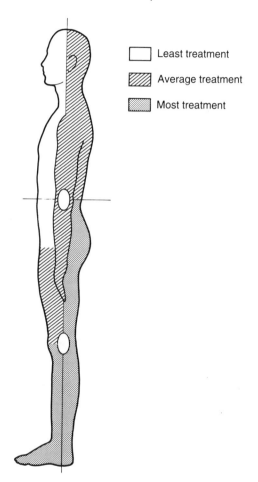

Least treatment

Average treatment

Most treatment

Figure 8.1 Areas of electrical conductivity of the body.

usually combine the point finding with treatment of the acupoint when located. Those who do not wish to use invasive methods can treat the point by leaving the probe *in situ* or attaching a surface electrode to the area located and the electro-stimulation can be applied without piercing the skin. There are drawbacks to this method of locating points. The skin of the patient may be too dry, in which case there is poor conductivity, or too moist which tends to blur the potential electrical responses, thus giving false readings. There are now more sophisticated instruments being marketed, which adjust for different skin conditions. Some practitioners work entirely on the measurement of the electrical potential between the different sides of the body and the perceived energy of the acupoints, to diagnose energy imbalance. This is usually done at meridian points at the wrists and ankles. Comparisons are then made between the readings and a treatment plan formulated based on these findings.

Another way to treat the acupoints non-invasively is to use a laser application. This is discussed in Chapter 11.

8.3 TO STIMULATE PAIN COPING MECHANISMS

Extensive research carried out on animals has shown that there is a specific response of the pain mechanism to different electrical frequencies. Practitioners can decide whether a long-term effect on pain is required, or whether a more immediate response is needed. For example, 2–4 Hz frequency using needles close to the area of pain works through the endorphin system and acts on the midbrain, spinal cord and pituitary–hypothalamus. This raises the pain threshold and gives a continuing relief of pain after the stimulation is withdrawn. Its effect is cumulative. 100–150 Hz frequency on the other hand activates part of the spinal cord and midbrain bypassing the endorphin system and thus gives an immediate analgaesic effect (Pomeranz and Stux, 1991). Some stimulators can deliver a combination of low and high frequency giving both long and short-term anaesthetic effect.

8.4 TO SUPPLY AND SEDATE ACUPOINTS

It is important to know the effect on the acupoint of stimulation with electrical stimuli. The basic principles of 'supplying' and 'reducing' the point are still relevant to treatment. Low (2–10 Hz) frequency tonifies but if applied over long periods, e.g. 30 minutes, it sedates. High (100 Hz) frequency sedates. Care needs to be taken when stimulating the needles. It is very easy to over stimulate and to cause sedation of a point inadvertently.

8.4.1 The stimulator

There are many machines which gives a variety of frequencies from which to choose for needle stimulation. A summary of the most useful attributes to look for in a stimulator is given below.

(a) Voltage

Should be adjustable 5–20 volts, the range mainly used being 5 to 10 volts. The power source can be either from the mains or by using dry batteries. The latter power source is more convenient and safer.

(b) Frequency

This should be adjustable from 1 to 150 Hz for low and higher frequency delivery.

(c) Types of current

i. Dispersed regular (2 Hz) tonifies and raises the pain threshold.
ii. Dense regular (50–200 Hz) sedates, but this is not long-lasting. The patient will quickly become tolerant to this frequency and the intensity will have to be increased to maintain the effect.
iii. Dense dispersal. This delivers short periods of dispersed regular alternately with dense regular. This is the most universally useful waveform.

(d) Design

The controls on the electro-stimulator should be large enough to enable the operator to finely adjust the intensity of the treatment so as to ensure patient comfort at all times.

A basic apparatus capable of giving the above waveforms need not be very elaborate. The simpler the display the better is the understanding of what is being delivered to the patient.

There are many machines which give elaborate computerized treatments for different identified disorders. Purchase of such machines must be a matter of personal judgement of the practitioner.

8.4.2 Duration and intensity of treatment with electro-stimulation

Some areas of the body are more conductive than others (Figure 8.1), e.g. the lower back and legs (other than knees) are less conductive and would need more stimulation. The posterior thorax,

skull and arms (other than elbows) have average conductivity
and the anterior aspect of the thorax and skull as well as the
elbows and knees are highly conductive and thus require less
stimulation to achieve the chosen effect (Woollerton and McLean,
1979).

8.5 ELECTRO-ACUPUNCTURE ACCORDING TO VOLL

It should be mentioned that there is a school of thought that has
extended the scope of electro-acupuncture to include diagnosis of
energy at any acupoint. This method is known as electro-acupuncture according to Voll (EAP). The machine used for this
purpose is the EAV-Dermatron. This was developed by R. Voll of
Germany. It is based on the principle that an acupoint has a
higher electrical conductivity relative to the immediate surrounding skin area, and that in conditions of disease, there is usually a
further decrease in the resistance of that point. This in turn indicates that there is a blockage in the free flow of energy in that
meridian and a disorder present in the related organ. When an
imbalance in the acupoint is found the equilibrium is restored
by stimulating the acupoint or points. Improvement can be
measured objectively. The theory and practice of this diagnostic
and therapeutic technique is a topic that is not addressed in this
text.

8.6 GUIDELINES FOR USING ELECTRO-STIMULATION

There are various factors to be aware of when stimulating acupuncture needles with electrical impulses.

8.6.1 Situations when not to electrically stimulate the acupuncture needle

• The points GV 20 (*bahui*) and PC 6 (*neiguan*). There have been
  some reports of headaches resulting from stimulation of *bahui*
  and cardiac irregularity when *neiguan* is stimulated.
• All 'dangerous points' which are defined in TCM.
• Those patients who have a cardiac pacemaker.
• Patients who may have convulsions or epilepsy.
• During pregnancy.
• Non-cooperative, mentally sub-normal or over-anxious
  patients.

8.6.2 Connecting needles to the stimulator

Do not couple:

* a *yin* and *yang* point;
* a tonification and sedation point;
* points on either side of the body especially with patients who have any hypertensive/cardiac problems (Jayasuriya, 1979).

8.6.3 Technique of electro-acupuncture

Metal objects in the vicinity of the area to be treated should be removed. NB Metal fillings and internal prostheses, however, are not a contraindication.

The points are first located and the needles inserted as in normal acupuncture. The stimulator is checked to ensure that the setting is at zero before attaching the leads to the needles. The current is then slowly increased until the patient feels a tingling sensation. This should normally not be strong enough to cause muscle contraction, but if greater stimulation over a pair of points is needed then the current can be increased to a point where there is muscle contraction. It should be noted that this also means that the points stimulated in this way will undergo a marked 'sedation'.

All stimulation should be within the patient's tolerance threshold. A sudden surge of current could cause muscle spasm and involuntary movement resulting in bending or breaking the needles. It is good practice to stimulate proximal and distal points on the same channel with one pair of electrodes.

If the patient has an adverse response while treatment is in progress, i.e. fainting or excessive sweating, then the stimulation should be stopped immediately and the needles withdrawn.

8.7 CONCLUSIONS

The main advantage of electro-acupuncture is that less time is needed to achieve the required effect of acupuncture treatment. In a busy practice patients can be set up on treatment and left for a while while another patient can be seen.

The practice of using electrical stimulation of needles is one of personal choice. Those who choose this method frequently claim good results. It has been shown to be more effective in pain relief than either transcutaneous electrical nerve stimulation (TENS) or placebo (Lehmann *et al.*, 1986).

The principle of using different frequencies to stimulate the spinal cord, midbrain and hypothalamus–pituitary to give short and long-term pain relief has been shown to be effective. The intensity of the stimulation also affects the degree of analgesia in chronic pain. Mao *et al.* demonstrated that the level of platelet serotonin varied according to the intensity of electrostimulation given through needles placed in acupoints. The higher intensity, which caused muscle twitching, resulted in higher platelet serotonin in chronic pain subjects and also gave more effective pain relief (Mao *et al.*, 1980).

However, non-invasive techniques must be used when skin penetration is not tolerated by the patient or permitted in 'local' codes of practice.

REFERENCES

He Lianfang (1987) Review Article. Involvement of endogenous opioid peptides in acupuncture analgesia. *Pain*, **31**, 99–121.

Jayasuriya, A. (1979) *Clinical Acupuncture* (Seventh Edition), Medicina Alternativa International, Sri Lanka.

Lehmann, T.R., Russell, D.W., Spratt, H.C., King Liu, Y., Fairchild, M.L., and Christensen, S. (1986) 'Efficacy of electroacupuncture and TENS in the rehabilitation of chronic low back pain patients'. *Pain*, **26**, 277–290.

Mao, W., Ghia, J.N., Scott, D.S., Duncan, G.H., and Gregg, J.M. (1980) High versus low intensity acupuncture analgesia for treatment of chronic pain: Effect on platelet serotonin. *Pain*, **8**, 331–342.

Pomeranz, B. and Stux, G. (1991) Scientific basis of acupuncture, in *Basics of Acupuncture*, Springer Verlag, Berlin, Heidelberg, New York, London, Paris, Tokyo, Hong Kong, Barcelona, Chapter 2.

Woollerton, H. and McLean, C.J. (1979) *Acupuncture Energy in Health and Disease*, Thorsons Publishers Ltd, Wellingborough, Northants, Chapter 8.

FURTHER READING

Chaitow, L. (1983) *The Acupuncture Treatment of Pain*, Thorsons Publishers, Wellingborough, Northants.

9

Transcutaneous electrical nerve stimulation (TENS)

9.1 HISTORY

This modality has been known to be used as far back as 2000 years ago. Records have been found dating back to Roman times which describe the touching of an electrical fish as being efficacious in painful conditions.

Rather more recently the beneficial effect of electrical stimulation on pain has been widely researched. The increased knowledge of the different substances that are released into the system in response to pain has enabled researchers to differentiate the response to high and low frequency electrical stimulation. The efficacy of the various frequencies were worked out largely as a result of electrically stimulating acupuncture needles for anaesthesia in operative procedures.

In the 1960s in China, acupuncture anaesthesia was being pioneered. Initially the needles were inserted and stimulated manually. The electrical frequency of this method is calculated to be about 4–6 Hz. This was not practical in a busy operating theatre and another method of mechanical stimulation of the needles needed to be found. The solution was electrical stimulation. The needles were inserted into the acupoints and then wired to the stimulator using crocodile clips to connect the leads to the acupuncture needle handles. The success of this method of analgesia was then carried into general practice and extended for the relief of chronic pain. The further development of this knowledge has been to develop a non-invasive method of applying stimuli through the acupoints without using manual techniques.

TENS is now used widely in clinical practice for the relief of acute and chronic pain.

9.2 DIFFERENT WAYS OF APPLYING TENS

There are various methods which can be used in the application of TENS treatment.

- Local to the painful area.
- Along the nerve supply, e.g. sciatic nerve in back and leg pain.
- In the painful dermatome.
- On acupoints.

9.2.1 Local to the painful area

This method uses the electrical stimulus through the skin to activate type II and type III afferents (high threshold muscle sensory nerve fibres) which then send neural messages to the spinal cord (or brain) where neurochemicals and hormones are released. This can give good relief of pain but does not utilize the extra-rich neural supply that is present in the area of the acupoints.

9.2.2 Along the line of the nerve affected

An example of this method could be when pain is felt in the lateral aspect of the leg. This would mean placing the pads over the head of the fibula where the lateral popliteal nerve emerges from the popliteal fossa and distally along the path of the lateral popliteal nerve.

9.2.3 In the painful dermatome

This is utilizing the afferent response as in 9.2.1 but with a stronger focus on one nerve.

One electrode could be placed at the level of the nerve root and the other on the corresponding dermatome where the pain is experienced, e.g. in femoral nerve pain one pad would be placed at the side of the upper lumbar vertebrae (L1, L2, L3) and the second pad placed anterior on the thigh or groin or over the most painful area.

The three methods above are all based on the present state of Western knowledge of the physiology of pain.

9.2.4 Placing the electrodes over acupoints

There are two reasons to use this method.

- To give more effective pain relief.
- To stimulate acupoints which in traditional Chinese medicine have a known specific effect.

(a) To give more effective pain relief

The nature and existence of acupoints has been discussed in Chapter 7. Research has shown that many acupoints coincide with trigger points which, when touched or probed, give relief of pain both locally and in areas distal to the point (Travell and Simons, 1983). Other researchers have identified many different nerve stuctures in the vicinity of the acupoints which if stimulated will initiate the pain-relieving mechanisms of the spinal cord and midbrain. Research has shown that the effect on pain can be greater than that of electrically stimulating needles inserted in acupoints (Cheng and Pomeranz, 1987).

Personal experience has proved that quite startling results can be achieved with this non-invasive modality, e.g. for temporo-mandibular joint (TMJ) pain. Point selection for this condition could be LI 4 *hegu* as a distal point with special effect on facial pain and ST 7 *xiaguan*, local to the TMJ (an actual case is described in Part Three).

(b) To stimulate acupoints which in traditional Chinese medicine (TCM) have a known specific effect

An example of this can be found in the study investigating the use of TENS on PC 6 *neiguan*, to enhance the effect of anti-emetic drugs used in patients who have cancer (McMillan and Dundee, 1991).

The application of TENS to acupoints using traditional knowledge can also be an effective way to treat a patient when insertion of needles is not possible or when a regular stimulation of acupoints is desirable between treatment sessions. For example, pain in the buttock and area of the thigh over the tensor fascia lata. Here the rule of acupuncture which advocates the use of the *ho* point on a meridian together with a point along the same channel can be used. Thus, GB 30 *huantiao* (local point in the gluteus maximus) and GB 34 *yanglinguan* (just below the head of the fibula) can be stimulated.

Lower back pain
Pain affecting the lower back without referred symptoms can be tackled in two ways.

* Electrodes placed on BL 24 *qihaishu* bilaterally (which is a specific point for the lumbar spine).
* Electrodes placed one over BL 24 *qihaishu* and one over the *ho* point of the bladder meridian BL 40 *weizhong*. Using a dual channel machine, a 4-pole method can be used to stimulate the right and left side simultaneously.

If local lumbar pain is combined with a kidney *xu* condition, using a dual channel stimulator, the electrodes could be placed on BL 23 *shenshu* in combination with BL 24 *qihaishu*.

When a patient needs to have continuing treatment between clinical visits, it is not always possible to re-apply the electrodes to the back. It is difficult to secure electrodes correctly on oneself especially if there is any restriction in shoulder movement. In these cases the knowledge of TCM is useful. LI 4 *hegu* is one of the most effective points for low back pain. Personal experience has shown that stimulation of this point with TENS can give some relief of low back pain and is relatively easy to apply.

Peripheral circulatory problems
There are some clinicians who are advocating the use of TENS for peripheral circulatory disorders. Kaada in 1986 reported on the treatment of ischaemia and chronic ulceration by TENS. More recently Dr G. Gibb, Consultant Rheumatologist, New Zealand (1991) spoke of regular treatment by TENS on LI 4 *hegu* to boost circulation.

There are some athletes who have 20 minutes strong stimulation of LI 4 *hegu* prior to training/competition in order to enhance athletic performance.

Personal experience in rheumatology of using LI 4 *hegu* for chronic leg ulcers, in this way, has been encouraging in the few cases encountered to date.

9.3 TECHNIQUE OF APPLICATION

9.3.1 Electrodes

The basic electrode is small and pliable and made of electocon-
ductive carbon-filled vinyl (2 × 3 cm). A simple water-based gel
is spread over the electrode. This should be sufficient to cover the
surface but not to spread beyond the margin of the electrode
when applied to the skin. A simple way to achieve an even application is to put the gel on the centre of one electrode and then
press the second electrode against it, moving the gel around until
evenly distributed on both electrodes. Securing to the skin can be
easily accomplished with a hyposensitive tape. The other, much
less messy, method is to use adhesive gel pads which adhere to
the skin and electrode without further adhesive being necessary.
These have a limited life and can become expensive in the long
term although the convenience and saving of time must not be
overlooked. Finally, there are the electrodes which are self-adhe-
sive and disposable; these are the simplest of all to use.

It is very important that pressure is evenly distributed over the
electrodes, as areas of uneven pressure could result in skin burns
at the edge of the pad where there is a high concentration of
current. The size of the pads also decides the comfortable intensity of the stimulation. Smaller pads concentrate the current and
therefore less stimulation can be achieved in the area. Larger pads
(6 × 6 cm) allow for a larger area of skin to be stimulated and thus
the intensity is spread and the higher intensities can be more
comfortably achieved which will allow sufficient stimulation
of the type III muscle fibres, which in turn stimulate the various biophysical responses of the pain mechanisms. A pad larger
than this would increase the area to such an extent as to cause a
drop in the current density and deep muscle fibres will not be
activated.

9.3.2 Machines

There are an infinate number of TENS machines on the market.
When considering the best for universal treatment, one would do
well to bear in mind the frequencies which give the best pain
relief. 2–4 Hz stimulates 5HT which gives a long-term relief of

pain, whereas 80–150 Hz stimulates the mechanism which has an immediate effect on pain. At the same time one needs to be aware of the use of TENS for stimulating acupoints for non-painful disorders.

A typical specification could be:

Pulse shape: bi-directional square pulse shape with fast rise time to overcome skin resistance.

Pulse amplitude: 0.55 mA constant current output into 1000 ohms.

Pulse rate: continuous mode, pulse frequency 2–100 Hz. Disperse and dense mode, disperse 2 Hz and dense 15–100 Hz. Burst mode, intermittent trains of impulses at 2 bursts per second, impulse frequency 15–100 Hz.

Machines that can deliver a variable stimulation prevent habituation and are more effective in relieving pain (Cheng and Pomeranz, 1987).

9.3.3 Optimum time for treatment for the relief of pain

There has been until recently a belief that treatment with TENS needs to be applied over long periods of time in order to achieve relief of pain. Periods of up to 8–10 hours have been suggested. However, recent research has shown that continuous stimulation using TENS of over an hour duration has the effect of stimulating anti-opiates which counter the pain relieving effect of treatment (Han, 1991).

It is now recommended that treatment be intermittent with not more than 1 hour allowed at one time for the stimulator to be used. This should ensure that the mechanisms producing the endorphins are not overstimulated.

Another technique is to vary the points that are stimulated, e.g. LI 4 *hegu* can be stimulated on alternate sides thus giving the type III muscle fibres periodic rest from activation.

Contraindication for treatment are the same as those for electro-acupuncture.

9.4 CONCLUSIONS

The practice of using TENS machines is widespread. They are small and portable and are under the control of the patient. This is psychologically good because it involves them in their own treatment. The nature of the electrical impulse is important. To achieve optimum effect the stimulation should be strong and variable to avoid habituation.

It could be said that in a patient with long-term painful disease, a TENS machine pays for itself by the saving made on prescriptions for analgesics.

REFERENCES

Cheng, R.S.S. and Pomeranz, B. (1987) Electrotherapy of chronic musculoskeletal pain: comparison of electroacupuncture and acupuncture-like transcutaneous nerve stimulation. *Clin. J. Pain*, 2, 143–149.
Han, C.S. (1991) 'The neural pathway mediating acupuncture analgesia'. Lecture delivered at The Fourth International Congress on Traditional and Modern Acupuncture, Gold Coast, Australia.
Gibb, G. (1991) Diagnostic and clinical manipulation of bio-energetic systems. The 4th Australian International Congress of Medical Acupuncture.
Kaada, B. (1986) Treatment of peripheral ischaemia and chronic ulceration by TENS. *Acupuncture Medicine*, 3, 30.
McMillan, O.M. and Dundee, J.W. (1991) The role of transcutaneous electrical stimulation of neiguan anti-emetic acupuncture point in controlling sickness after cancer chemotherapy. *Physiotherapy*, 77(7), 499–501.
Travell, J. and Simons, D. (1983) Myofascial pain and dysfunction. *The Trigger Point Manual*, William and Wilkins, Baltimore.

10

Trigger point acupuncture

One of the main problems which is met by a physiotherapist in clinical practice is musculo-skeletal pain. There are many ways in which this can be addressed.

Historically, massage was widely used to alleviate painful symptoms. Tender nodules were identified within the muscles and kneaded. These local nodules were acutely painful to palpate but the relief after massage was felt not only in the area of tenderness but in areas distal to the treated painful nodule. These have subsequently been identified as trigger points.

In 1938 a report was published which identified referred pain arising from muscle (Kellgren, 1938). He showed that injecting saline deep into muscle tissue after first anaesthetizing the superficial area induced pain distal to the area infiltrated. He also found that sometimes the most severe pain was felt at the referred site rather than in the local area of the muscle which was injected. Areas or nodules which were acutely tender were identified and then injected with novocaine. There was substantial pain relief not only in the area injected but in areas where pain was felt distal to the 'trigger point area'.

There were further experiments carried out using different substances to inject the trigger points including saline, which proved to be as effective as local anaesthetic. The conclusion was drawn that it was the penetration of the needle into the hypersensitive point which was the significant factor in the relief of myofascial pain.

There have been further studies into how this pain is referred and many theories put forward. Experimental work has shown that there does not appear to be a fixed pattern in the referral of the pain. Many researchers have found, however, that the trigger points identified in different subjects are often to be found in similar locations. The spatial distribution of trigger points which were identified by several researchers was compared to the location of acupoints (Melzack and Stillwell, 1977) and there was found to be a 71% correlation.

10.2 IDENTIFYING THE TRIGGER POINT

The true trigger point is acutely painful. It is an actual nodule or tight band of tissue in the muscle and it is relatively easy to palpate. There is now an established core of clinical experience which has identified specific areas of referred pain caused by trigger points in the muscles. The following are just two examples of syndromes that could respond to trigger point acupuncture.

10.2.1 Anterior shoulder pain

An extension strain can cause pain felt in the anterior of the shoulder joint. It sometimes radiates down to the thumb and first two fingers of the hand via the antero-lateral aspect of the arm and can cause sleep to be disturbed when the patient lies on either side.

If the patient has limited medial rotation of the shoulder and describes a repeated strain, e.g. reaching backwards as could happen when picking up items from the back seat of a car, or falling backwards on the outstretched arm, then a strain of the infra spinatus could be the cause. The site of trigger points in this muscle is consistently found below the spine of the scapula.

To palpate for trigger points in the muscle the arm should be flexed and adducted across the chest, putting the infra spinatus on a stretch. The area of the infra spinatus fossa just below the spine of the scapula should be explored with the fingers of both hands using a probing firm pressure. The whole of the muscle should be palpated and areas of exquisite tenderness noted.

10.2.2 Low back pain

The sites for trigger points are not so predictable in this area as in the shoulder and cervical region.

Examination is carried out initially with the patient in a prone position. The muscles should be palpated by placing the hands over the area and gently kneading the muscles. The area from T10 level down to the iliac crest can be covered moving the hands parallel to each other down the spine and then extending outward so that all the muscles have been felt between the iliac crest and the rib cage. The search continues into the gluteii and the lateral aspect of the hips when the patient then has to be examined on alternate sides. Finally the abdomen should be examined in the supine position and the medial aspect of the thigh and groin. Trigger points identified in the pubic area, especially where the adductor muscles are attached, can give rise to vaginal and scrotal pain as well as pain in the low back in a sitting posture. Areas of acute tenderness can be found either localized to one point in an otherwise normal muscle or in tight fibrous bands that the fingers can slide over (Baldry, 1989).

10.3 TECHNIQUE OF TRIGGER POINT ACUPUNCTURE

When the patient is seen for the first time, the response to acupuncture is unknown and over-treating the trigger points can exacerbate pain.

Having identified the trigger points they now have to be desensitized. The acupuncture needle is put into the skin immediately superficial to the trigger point penetrating the upper dermal area only. The needle is left *in situ* for about 30 seconds only. It is gently rotated and the patient asked if there is any sensation felt where the needle is placed. If the answer is 'Yes', a further period of 30 seconds is allowed and the test repeated. When there is no sensation felt, the needle is removed and the trigger point palpated. There should be relief of local pain. If there is still tenderness felt, a further needling is necessary in the same way as described above.

All the trigger points identified in this way must be desensitized. If one is missed there is incomplete relief of referred pain. Several trigger points can be treated at the same time.

On subsequent treatments the sensitivity is known and the needles can be left for longer periods if indicated.

10.4 PRECAUTIONS TO BE TAKEN

All the precautions applying to acupuncture apply to this form of treatment.

10.4.1 Patient's history

It is important to get an adequate history from the patient so that any sinister cause of pain can be eliminated. Relief of pain without first ascertaining the underlying cause can in some cases prove dangerous if the underlying cause of pain is due to malignancy and vital diagnosis delayed.

10.4.2 Dangerous areas

Care must be taken when treating points around the chest wall as there is a danger of pneumothorax should the needles penetrate the pleura.

10.4.3 Delayed reaction

Sometimes following treatment there is sudden and complete relief of pain accompanied by a feeling of euphoria. The patient should be warned that a return of severe pain may be experienced after several hours. This situation should be avoided by adhering to the technique described above of leaving the needles *in situ* for a minimal period only.

10.5 DISADVANTAGES

The first disadvantage of this method of acupuncture is purely a practical one. The technique of treating the points and constantly testing them for sensitivity requires the constant presence of the practitioner. This does limit the number of patients that can be treated during a clinic session.

The second disadvantage is that it is operative only on relieving pain without ascertaining the underlying cause. A full case history which includes an analysis of the lifestyle and occupation of the patient can establish the cause of the musculo-skeletal pain. A programme of exercise and postural advice can then be worked out to complement the acupuncture treatment.

10.6 CONCLUSIONS

Trigger point acupuncture is an extremely useful technique for the relief of musculo-skeletal pain. Its effectiveness is dependent on scrupulous location of all the trigger points and careful stimulation of the needles when *in situ*.

REFERENCES

Baldry, P.E. (1989) Low back pain, in *Acupuncture, Trigger Points and Musculoskeletal Pain*. Churchill Livingstone, Edinburgh, London, Melbourne, New York.

Kellgren, J.H. (1938) A preliminary account of referred pain arising from muscle. *Br. Med. J.*, **1**, 325–327.

Melzack, R. and Stillwell, D.M. (1977) Trigger points and acupuncture points for pain: correlations and implications. *Pain*, **3**, 3–23.

11

The use of lasers in acupuncture

In this section the way in which a laser works is described and its use in both simple pain relief and other disorders will be discussed.

11.1 HISTORY

The word LASER is derived from the initial letters of the following words: Light Amplification by Stimulated Emission of Radiation. In 1960 Dr. Theodore Maiman working in California was first to produce a powerful pulse of intense light in the red part of the spectrum using a ruby crystal. In the following year two gases were mixed, namely helium (He) and neon (Ne), and this HeNe laser also produced a red light. Alongside this development came the infrared laser, which was based on an yttrium aluminium garnet crystal doped with neodymium. This was the YAG or Nd:YAG laser.

These lasers with modifications have remained the principle lasers used in surgery and medicine today. The practice of laser surgery is well established, especially where very delicate techniques are required, such as in ophthalmology.

11.2 LASERS

11.2.1 The components of a laser

(a) The laser medium

Whether the heart of the laser is formed by a crystal, or a mixture of gases such as HeNe, it is referred to as the laser medium.

Some lasers combine the visible red beam of a HeNe laser and the invisible infrared beam from CO_2 and Nd:YAG lasers. The visible light is used as an aiming beam for the invisible beam.

Semiconductors, such as gallium aluminium arsenide (GaAlAs), are also used for media. It is this source that is most significant to practitioners using lasers for acupuncture, because it forms the basis of one of the most effective applicators of Low Level Laser Therapy (LLLT).

The wavelength of the laser beam is dependent on the atomic and molecular composition of the medium, and the interaction between the medium and energy source.

(b) The resonating cavity

The cavity consists of the medium with two mirrors placed at right angles to the axis of the medium at either end of the cavity. These mirrors are coated to allow only one particular wavelength to be reflected and allowing all the other parts of the spectrum to pass through. The mirrors are not identical. One at the rear of the resonating cavity will be 100% reflective while the other only partly reflective and it is the latter mirror that emits the laser beam.

(c) The energy source

To create laser emissions, energy must be introduced to the laser medium and converted to light, or photon energy. The added energy could be light energy from a flash lamp, electrical energy passing through the medium, or the energy resulting from chemical reaction within the medium. The energy to activate the laser emission is called **pumping**.

If any of the above described components is lacking in the system there will be no laser emission. The design and placing of all the various components must be precise in order that the pumping energy source can successfully activate the laser emission.

11.2.2 Wavelength

Electromagnetic radiation travels in discrete particles of energy called **photons** or **quanta**. These particles follow regular wavelike pathways. By measuring the distance between one 'peak' and the

next along the waveform of a particular group of particles, the
wavelength of these particles is found The waveform determines
if it is visible or not.

A laser emits light at a specific discrete single wavelength and
is of a pure colour, unlike a domestic strip light which emits a
wide spectrum of colours resulting in a whitish light.

11.2.3 Phase

An incandescent light source such as a normal domestic light
emits photons which fly off in random directions without any
conformity, whereas the laser emits the photons in one unified
direction. The resulting beam has little divergence. The tendency
for the photons in the laser beam to remain almost parallel is
called **collimation**.

11.2.4 Coherence

The sum of monochromaticity, phase and collimation is called
coherence. Coherent laser beams can be focused to extremely
small spot sizes. This enables the practitioner to be extremely
accurate when treating acupoints.

11.2.5 Laser/tissue interaction

Experimental work has shown that there are interesting changes
which take place when injured tissues are exposed to LLLT. Mast
cells and macrophages can be stimulated to release growth factors
and other substances and there is a measurable increase in
fibroblasts and keratinocytes. There is also evidence of increased
uptake of calcium ions in the treated area (Dyson, 1991). This
effect has significance on the rate of cellular activity and healing
of lesions.

Further effects include increased vasodilatation. The non-thermal effect which is achieved by low level lasers in the target tissue
has been shown to cause a rise in temperature of maximum 1°C.
The conclusion therefore must be that the laser stimulates
through its electromagnetic energy.

11.3 THE LOW LEVEL LASER THERAPY UNIT

The laser apparatus that is used by acupuncturists is the Low
Level Laser Therapy unit (LLLT). This is sometimes called a soft

laser. The first lasers used therapeutically were all in the visible red range (632 nm) from a helium neon source.

The penetration of the 'visible' laser is 0.8 mm directly with an additional 3 mm corona around the beam as revealed by histological staining (Harrison, 1989).

Later infrared lasers with 904 nm wavelength and 5–10 mW intensity generated from gallium arsenide diodes were also manufactured. Now the latest devices are produced giving 780 nm and 10–15 mW intensity and it is possible to have interchangeable laser applicators giving visible and non-visible beams generated from the same apparatus.

11.4 LASER ACUPUNCTURE

The development of laser stimulation of acupoints has a similar history to that of electro-acupuncture. It is used in two ways.

11.4.1 Anaesthetic effect

It began to be used in lieu of needles on acupoints to achieve an anaesthetic effect. It was non-invasive and therefore eliminated the possibility of infection.

It is now found to be most successful in maxillary surgery and dental procedures. Exposure to laser of only 5 minutes on facial points is found to be optimum and then throughout the operative procedure LI 4 (*hegu*) is irradiated (Ohshiro and Calderhead, 1988).

If an anaesthetic effect is required, exposure of 5 minutes is not uncommon. In acupuncture terms this would sedate the point.

11.4.2 Stimulating acupoints in a therapeutic treatment programme

In China, laser stimulation is used in treating children, as it can be applied to the acupoints without causing discomfort. This practice has been much extended in the West and many practitioners use only a laser source for acupuncture in their clinical practice.

In laser stimulation it is not normal to achieve *deqi* but there still seems to be an effect on the acupoint. In the former Soviet Union there was a great deal of work to establish optimum dosage of laser to produce an effect through the acupoint. Using a HeNe laser with an output of 25 mW, radiation of 5–10 seconds was found to 'supply' and 30–120 seconds application to 'sedate' the point.

The dosages are now expressed in joules/mm^2. This is worked out by the following formula:

$$\text{Joules/mm}^2 = \text{Output (mW)} \times \text{Time (s)} \times \text{Area of beam (mm}^2).$$

For example, given a HeNe laser of 0.79 cm^2 (beam) and an output of 3 mW, the saturation dosage for ear points would be 0.14 J/mm^2 and this would be achieved by treating the point for 1 minute (Harrison, 1989).

Another factor to take into account when using a laser for acupuncture treatment is that the depth of penetration is limited and effective treatment of the *ho* points or deeper abdominal points is very doubtful. However the more peripheral points on the hands and feet can be effectively treated, but the timing of the application is dependent on the strength of the laser.

PRECAUTIONS:

1. It is important to protect the eyes from direct laser exposure and it is advisable for the patient to wear special protective goggles. The practitioner should also be thus protected, but the vision is greatly impaired by such goggles and observing a technique which does not direct the beam directly towards oneself should be sufficient.
2. Some regions have by-laws concerning LLLT and these should be ascertained before purchasing equipment.

11.5 CONCLUSIONS

In laser therapy the indications for treatment are the same as for conventional acupuncture. The potential of this therapy is enormous. To be able to effectively treat a condition without piercing skin removes the risk of cross infection and is less traumatic for the patient.

In reality it is probably most effective on the more superficial points, e.g. *tsing* and ear points, as penetration of the beam is only 2–5 mm, although there is some indirect effect deeper in the tissues. It is a *yang* source of energy and would be more appropriate to use in deficiency of *yang* syndromes.

The shallow penetration will also enable *wei qi*, which runs subcutaneously, to be influenced. Patients sometimes state that they feel the effect of the laser far from the point of application, which would appear to confirm the hypothesis that the electromagnetic effects are transmitted in this way.

It is important, however, to validate the effects claimed for this therapy. Treating the acupoints in lieu of needles in the traditional sense can pose difficulties in timing the treatment, if a specific 'supplying' or 'sedating' effect is required.

REFERENCES

Dyson, M. (1991) Lecture: 'Cellular effects of phototherapy', Electrotherapy Conference, The Royal National Hospital for Rheumatic Diseases, Bath.

Harrison, A. (1989) Laser acupuncture, a review. *Br. J. Ac.*, **12**(2), 20–2.

Ohshiro, T. and Calderhead, R.G. (1988) *Low Level Laser Therapy, A Practical Introduction*, John Wiley and Sons.

12

Auricular therapy

12.1 INTRODUCTION

12.1.1 History

This chapter is included in Part Two of this book because much of the development of auricular therapy has taken place in the West, although it is now extensively practised in China.

There are records dating back to 200–300 BC describing the ear not as an isolated organ, but part of the *zang/fu* system. The meridians of the *fu* organs are identified as entering different parts of the ear but not the *zang* meridians. These are represented indirectly through their connections with the *fu* meridians.

In the West treatment of the ear is documented as far back as 1637, when Zactus Lusitanus reported good results from cauterizing the ear to relieve sciatic pain. Dr Ruther in 1950 also reported success in sciatic pain by cauterizing the helix of the ear. This technique is also used in China today, although the heating is done using a moxa roll.

Dr. P.M.F. Nogier first became aware of the effect of auricular therapy when patients described treatment using cautery in the ear. Over a period of twenty years from the 1950s to the 1970s he mapped out various areas on the ear which seem to relate to parts of the body and to affect the emotions. This was independent to TCM theory. In this chapter only the TCM approach will be addressed but the techniques described are equally applicable to the Nogier points (Figure 12.1). The anatomy, technique of locating and treating points will be described as well as the part auricular therapy can play in a treatment programme.

12.1.2 The anatomy of the auricle

There are two aspects to the anatomy of the auricle.

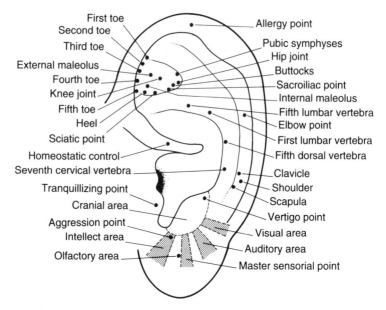

Figure 12.1 Location of a selection of Dr Nogier's ear acupoints.

(a) Anatomical features: There are distinct landmarks (Figure 12.2), which enable the practitioner to locate the points in particular areas.
(b) The imagined shape of a human fetus curled up head downwards (Figure 12.3) enables the practitioner to understand why the points relate to certain parts of the body.

(a) Anatomical features (Figure 12.2)

1. Helix: inverted rim of the auricle.
2. Crus helicis: prominent oblique ridge, at antero-inferior end of the helix.
3. Auricular tubercle (Darwin's tubercle): the small projection in the free margin of the helix.
4. Cauda helicis: the inferior end of the helix at its junction with the lobule.
5. Antihelix: a prominent semicircular ridge lying parallel to the main curve of the helix, it divides into the superior and inferior crus.
6. Triangular fossa (deltoid): the depression between the two crura of the antihelix.

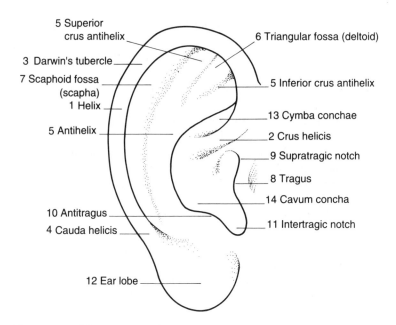

Figure 12.2 The anatomy of the ear from the Western aspect.

5 Superior crus antihelix

3 Darwin's tubercle

7 Scaphoid fossa (scapha)

1 Helix

5 Antihelix

10 Antitragus

4 Cauda helicis

12 Ear lobe

6 Triangular fossa (deltoid)

5 Inferior crus antihelix

13 Cymba conchae

2 Crus helicis

9 Supratragic notch

8 Tragus

14 Cavum concha

11 Intertragic notch

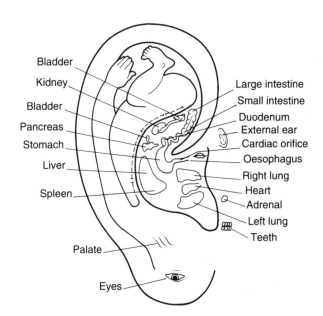

Bladder
Kidney
Bladder
Pancreas
Stomach
Liver
Spleen
Palate
Eyes

Large intestine
Small intestine
Duodenum
External ear
Cardiac orifice
Oesophagus
Right lung
Heart
Adrenal
Left lung
Teeth

Figure 12.3 The anatomy of the ear from the Chinese aspect, indicating the form of an inverted fetus with different parts of the ear associated with different organs of the body.

7. Scapha: the trough-shaped depression between the helix and antihelix.
8. Tragus: the petal-shaped projection over the entrance to the meatus.
9. Supratragic notch: the depression between the crus helicis and the upper border of the tragus.
10. Antitragus: A small tubercle opposite the tragus and inferior to the antihelix.
11. Intertragic notch: the depression between the tragus and the antitragus.
12. Lobule: the lower part of the auricle where the cartilage is absent.
13. Cymba conchae: the concha superior to the helix crus.
14. Cavum conchae: the concha inferior to the helix crus.
15. Orifice of the external auditory meatus: the opening is shielded by the tragus.

12.1.3 Nerve supply

The nerve supply is very rich, derived from the following:

- auriculo-temporal nerve;
- great auricular nerve;
- lesser occipital nerve;
- auricular branch of the vagus nerve;
- auriculo-temporal branch of the trigeminal nerve;
- branches of the glosso-pharyngeal and facial nerves;
- sympathetic and parasympathetic fibres.

12.1.4 Blood supply

This is derived from:

- branches of the middle meningeal artery;
- branch of the artery of the pterygoid canal;
- anterior tympanic artery;
- deep auricular artery;
- stylomastoid branch of the posterior auricular artery;
- auricular branches of the superficial auricular artery.

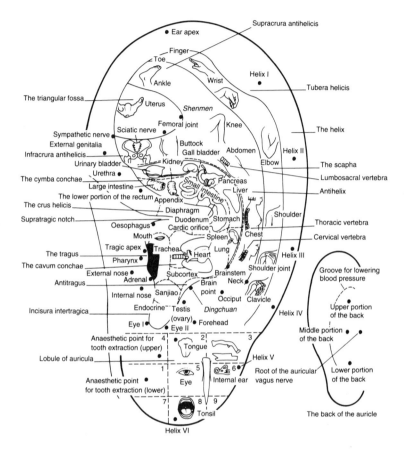

Figure 12.4 Location of acupoints on the ear, according to traditional Chinese medicine.

12.2 AREAS AND POINTS ON THE ANTERIOR OR *YANG* SURFACE (Figure 12.4)

12.2.1 The ear lobe

This represents the face. It is divided into nine treatment areas:

- Area 1 and area 4: anaesthetic points for tooth extraction and analgesia points for toothache.

- Area 1 represents teeth of lower jaw and area 4 the teeth of the upper jaw.
- Area 2: the middle of this area represents the tongue. The upper part of the area represents the hard palate and the lower area the soft palate.
- Area 3: represents the jaws, the upper border the lower jaw and the lower border the upper jaw.
- Area 5: this is in the middle of the ear lobe and represents the eye. There are also two other eye areas (eye I and eye II) either side of the intertragic notch. Eye I is indicated for astigmatism and eye II for glaucoma.
- Area 6: represents the inner ear. It is indicated for vertigo, dizziness, travel sickness, nausea and vomiting in pregnancy.
- Areas 7 and 9: have no identifiable points.
- Area 8: represents the tonsils and throat.
- There is an extra area lying between areas 5 and 6 called the facio-mandibular area. It is useful when treating facial paralysis, trigeminal neuralgia and sinusitis.

12.2.2 The tragus

Associated treatment areas are:

- Lateral aspect: At the centre of this aspect is the external nose area.
- Medial aspect: lying directly over the external auditory meatus is the pharynx area. Below this point is the internal nose area.
- Border of the tragus: on the free border at the lowest part is the adrenal point. Between the adrenal point and the external nose area is the hunger point (useful for treating obesity).

12.2.3 The antitragus

This corresponds to the head region.

(a) Lateral aspect of antitragus

- Forehead area: junction of area 2 of lobe with antitragus.
- Occiput area: superior part of antitragus.

- Parotid and temporal areas: lies between the forehead and occiput area.

(b) Free margin of antitragus

There are three important points to be found in this area.

- At the apex of the antitragus is the point *dinguan* (in Chinese this means soothing asthma). Needling this point during an acute attack of bronchial asthma can help to alleviate symptoms.
- Junction of the antitragus and antihelix: brain stem.
- Midway between *dinguan* and brain stem lies the brain point.

(c) Medial aspect of antitragus

The medial wall represents the sub-cortex. Testes or ovary are represented on the lower part of sub-cortex area. This area is adjacent to the endocrine area located in the intertragic notch.

12.2.4 The antihelix

This area represents the trunk. The lower part where the antihelix joins the antitragus is the neck area.

The inferior crus of the antihelix corresponds to the gluteal region and thigh. The superior crus of the antihelix corresponds to the lower extremity below and knee.

(a) The inferior crus of the antihelix

The posterior half of the inferior crus represents the buttock area with the hip joint area on the superior border adjacent to this area. The anterior part represents the lumbo-sacral plexus and the sciatic nerve area.

At the middle one-third of the upper groove of this area lies the constipation point.

At the junction between the superior and inferior crus lies the knee joint area.

(b) The superior crus of the antihelix

This represents the leg area with the toes uppermost.

12.2.5 The helix

There is a small prominence on the free margin of the helix at the junction of the upper and middle third of the helix, called Darwin's tubercle. It is significant in that it represents the *zang-fu* organs and is used as a homeostatic point.

12.2.6 The crus of the helix

This represents the diaphragm muscle.

The internal organs of the thorax are represented inferior to the crus of helix and the abdominal viscera superior to the crus of helix in the conchae.

Level with the crus of helix is the divide on the antihelix between the thoracic and lumbar spines, i.e. areas below this level represent the thoracic and neck areas and the areas above this level the lumbo-sacral area.

12.2.7 The scaphoid fossa (scapha)

The scapha represents the upper limb, the shoulder and clavicle area being at the level below the crus of helix. Above this level lies the elbow area which is level with the inferior end of the inferior crus of the antihelix. At the level of the inferior end of the superior crus is the wrist area. At the most superior part of the scapha is the area representing the fingers.

The line of the scapha continues downwards lying between the lobe and the antitragus. It represents the auditory functions and can be used for treating tinnitus, deafness, vertigo, and Ménière's disease.

12.2.8 The triangular fossa (deltoid fossa)

This is bounded on three sides by the helix, the superior crus of the antihelix (inferior border) and the inferior crus of the antihelix (superior border). One of the most frequently used points lies in this area.

(a) Ear point shenmen

This is located at the junction of the superior and inferior crus described above. It has a strong sedative effect as well as a wide spectrum of physiological effects. These include insomnia, hypertension, acute trauma and sciatica.

(b) Sympathetic point

This is at the junction of the helix and inferior crus. This is also a useful point for sympathetic pain, e.g. when pain is not primarily a result of motor nerve disorders.

(c) Hypertension point

This lies at the junction of the helix and superior crus. Useful for high blood pressure.

(d) Uterus point

This is at the midpoint between the hypertension and sympathetic point (in males this represents the prostate gland and seminal vesicle areas).

12.2.9 The cavum conchae

The deepest area represents the heart. This is posterior to the external auditory meatus. The posterior half of the line between the external auditory meatus and the heart area represents the trachea. The two lung areas are situated superior and inferior to the trachea and heart, the lower lung area representing the lung of the same side.

The area between the antitragus and tragus is divided into an upper half which is the area for the three body areas (thorax, abdomen, pelvis) and a lower half for the endocrine area.

The area at the lower rim of the external auditory meatus represents the upper abdominal wall and the area at the upper rim, the lower abdominal wall.

Immediately above and posterior to the external auditory meatus lies the mouth area. Between this area and the lower border of the crus helix is a secondary hunger point, which is used extensively in Western auricular therapy to treat obesity.

Posterior to the termination of the crus helix lies the stomach area and extending from this area to the mouth area is the area representing the oesophagus, just below the lower margin of the diaphragm. Between the stomach area and the antihelix is the spleen area.

12.2.10 The cymba conchae

The stomach area continues into the area superior to the crus helix. The organs are represented from posterior to anterior in the following order: duodenum, small intestine, appendix and large intestine and rectum.

Above the gastro-intestinal area in the cymba conchae lie the areas representing the liver, gall bladder, pancreas, kidney, urethra and urinary bladder.

There are some special factors to note when locating some areas.

* The pancreas is represented only in the left ear and the gall bladder in the right ear, both in the same location.
* Between the upper pole of the kidney and the small intestine area is the ascites point, which is useful for oedema.
* The external genitalia are represented in the helix above the urethra area.

12.3 THE MEDIAL, POSTERIOR OR *YIN* SURFACE

There is a groove on this surface, which corresponds to the scapha. This is specifically associated with lowering blood pressure. The rest of the *yin* surface is divided into three distinct areas horizontally. They are upper, middle and lower areas and are used in treating spinal disorders.

12.4 EXAMINATION OF THE EAR

This needs to be carefully carried out in order that the most effective points can be used in a treatment programme. There are three examination procedures which need to be completed before treatment is decided.

* Inspection. All parts of the ear should be looked at in order to identify areas which may have raised spots, peeling, or be inflamed. These are known as reactive areas and may have a bearing on the disorder being addressed.
* Tenderness. The tender or reactive points can be located by a

systematic palpation, which can be done with the handle end of an acupuncture needle or a matchstick.

- Electro-exploratory technique. A suitable electrical detector will show areas of reduced skin resistance, which may indicate a dysfunction of the corresponding organ.

12.5 SELECTING POINTS FOR TREATMENT IN AURICULAR THERAPY

1. Organ, e.g. stomach area for stomach disorders, lung point for bronchitis.
2. Coupled organ, e.g. spleen area for stomach disorders, large intestine for bronchitis.
3. Functions, e.g. high blood pressure, use hypertension point; obesity, use hunger point.
4. Relating function according to TCM, e.g. kidney area for arthritic conditions, lung area for skin problems, liver area for muscular or eye disorders.
5. Relating points according to the Theory of the Five Elements, e.g. lung point for stomach disorders when the pulse is over-full (lung is the son of Earth and therefore sedates). Lung point for anger (Metal controls Wood).
6. Disorder related points, e.g. point *dinchuan* for relieving asthma, *shenmen* for insomnia, sympathetic point for disorders of the sympathetic nervous system.
7. Western medicine associated points, e.g. point pancreas for diabetes mellitus, bladder point for urinary incontinence.
8. Reactive points. These are points that have been located through observation, palpation and electical reaction.
9. Endocrine point. This is very useful when the patient has been on long periods of medication and is especially indicated after prolonged steroid therapy, to alleviate withdrawal symptoms.
10. The tragus and *zang-fu* point. These are useful for general points to establish homeostasis in many disorders.

12.6 TECHNIQUE OF AURICULAR THERAPY

When the point has been located a needle can be inserted and left for 15–20 minutes as with body acupuncture points. A fine gauge (32 or 34 gauge) 1/2 inch needle is quite adequate for the purpose.

Stimulation of the needle is best carried out by electro-stimulation. Manual manipulation is too crude and may cause damage to the underlying cartilage. There should be a feeling of distension at the site of the needling as this indicates a good response.

There are three ways in which auricular therapy can be utilized.

12.6.1 Using ear points alone

The reasons for using only ear points are threefold:

1. The practitioner prefers to practise only auricular therapy.
2. The patient's site of pain may be inaccessible and therefore the appropriate ear point can be utilized.
3. Ear points can be used in helping various addictions. For example:
   (a) Nicotine: This is one of the hardest dependencies to cure. A great deal of psychological support is needed. Stimulating the lung point and ear *shenmen* with 5–10 Hz for 10–15 minutes is a good starting point. The acupuncture will only help to alleviate the withdrawal symptoms; the will-power of the patient must do the rest.

      Sadly there are many who revert back to the smoking habit even after several years of non-smoking. Personal experience is that those who begin to smoke in their early teens are rarely successful in giving up smoking.
   (b) Obesity: There has been less recorded success with this problem. Treatment should always be combined with dietary advice and psychological support. The resulting loss in weight could be said to be the result of the diet and counselling. However, the ear points to use are stomach, hunger and *shenmen* points.
   (c) Drug dependency: There have been many people who have become dependent on tranquillizers in recent years. Auricular therapy certainly has a part to play in these cases.

      Using ear points that can simulate the relaxing and calming effect of the drugs enables the dosage to be gradually reduced without too many withdrawal problems. The main point to use would be ear *shenmen*.

In all the addiction problems described above, body points can be used in the treatment sessions to boost the effect of the ear acupuncture.

A general treatment could be LI 4 (*hegu*) LR 3 (*taichong*) and ST 36 (*zusanli*). This has a calming and balancing effect on the body.

12.6.2 Using ear points in combination with body points

It is useful to combine auricular and body acupuncture to achieve a stronger effect in musculo-skeletal problems. For example:

1. In severe shoulder pain, the eyes of the shoulder plus LI 14 and 15 may be needled and this might be combined with inserting a needle in the shoulder point of the ear. This could be left *in situ* for 20 minutes or electro-stimulated. The frequency at which the electro-stimulator is set is variable. Bearing in mind the stimulation of the different pain mechanisms discussed in Chapters 7 and 8, a low or high frequency can be used. A press needle or non-invasive device could then be substituted which the patient can leave in place until the next treatment. This will continue (hopefully) the analgesic effect of the treatment.
2. In a problem of persistent leg pain, which has some circulation component, the sympathetic ear point can be stimulated as well as the local and distal points on the lower limb.
3. If the leg pain is sciatic in origin then the sciatic and buttock ear points can be used as well as the body points.
4. When there is an anxiety component to the patient's problem inclusion of ear point *shenmen* in the treatment should be considered.

12.6.3 Anaesthetic effect

Ear acupuncture is used for anaesthesia for extraction of teeth and also general surgical procedures. It is a useful technique to employ when it is not possible to put needles in body points.

12.7 PROBLEMS WHICH MAY ARISE AS A RESULT OF EAR ACUPUNCTURE

12.7.1 Infection

It is important first of all to be aware of the structure of the ear. There are large areas which have a very thin layer of skin covering cartilage which has no blood supply. Infection introduced into the cartilage can produce very severe results. Sometimes it has led to the amputation of the ear. The following precautions need to taken:

1. Extreme care in cleaning the ear prior to treatment is necessary and any infected areas should be avoided. To use single-use needles is essential unless there are adequate autoclaving facilities.
2. Do not penetrate the underlying cartilage.
3. Press needles can be inserted and left *in situ* for several days, but they need to be covered with a waterproof dressing to prevent any moisture entering the puncture site. Patients should be briefed carefully about possible adverse effects and told to come back immediately if there is any irritation or pain associated with the needle.

12.8 ACUPRESSURE

Many practitioners do not use needless in the ear but simply give acupressure either with massage or a probe. Press needles are replaced by a small ball-bearing or rape seed. This is secured with hypoallergic tape and left *in situ* between treatments. The patient is asked to press the wood chip/ball-bearing at least three times a day to stimulate the point.

When I was in Guangzhou (1983) they were well aware of the dangers of ear infection in auricular therapy and press needles were no longer used. Small chips of wood were used instead. Personal experience has demonstrated a good effect just by cutting small cubes of wood from a matchstick and securing them to the ear with hypoallergic tape.

12.9 ELECTRO-STIMULATION

12.9.1 Treatment using both ears

The needles should be placed *in situ* and wired to the electrotherapy machine, one ear wired to the negative and the other to the positive terminal.

12.9.2 Treatment involving only one ear

The needle should be wired to one terminal and the patient holds an electrode wired to the other terminal.

Stimulation should be for about 10–15 minutes. The strength of stimulation is governed by the patient, who should feel a mild burning sensation.

12.9.3 Treatment without needle insertion

This can be effected by placing a probe on the ear point while the patient holds the coupled electrode. Stimulation should be for 2–3 minutes (Huang, 1975).

12.10 CONCLUSIONS

Auricular therapy is a very useful modality to use in clinical practice. It has a wide range of therapeutic uses. It should be emphasized that only a brief outline of the TCM method of treatment of this complex modality has been given.

REFERENCE

Huang, H.L. (1975) *Ear Acupuncture: The Complete Text* by the Nanking Army Ear Acupuncture Team, Rodale Press, Inc., Book Division, Emmaus, Pennsylvania.

FURTHER READING

Jayasuriya, A. (1979) *Clinical Acupuncture*, the Acupuncture Foundation of Sri Lanka, Colombo.
Nogier, P.M.F. (1981) *Handbook on Auricular therapy*, Maisoneuve, 57160 Moulins le Metz, France.

Part Three

The Synthesis of Western Medicine and TCM in Treating Conditions met in Clinical Practice

Introduction

In previous sections the basic theories of TCM have been examined. In this section there will be discussion on how this knowledge can be used in a complete rehabilitation programme. The conditions addressed are those that are normally treated by physiotherapists.

It is important in clinical practice to be aware of the precautions and contraindications of using invasive techniques and to conform with the standards set by local legislation and by the practitioner's own professional society.

A practitioner may use part or all of the diagnostic procedures described in Part One, prior to formulating a treatment plan. Western diagnosis gives an established name to the presenting condition. Knowledge of traditional Chinese diagnosis can enable the practitioner to assess other underlying factors and address these as well.

When deciding how to treat the acupoints selected the principle of balancing the *yin* and *yang* energy should always be considered. If there is an excess of *yang* over *yin* this will be demonstrated in the underlying colour of the tongue, which will appear very bright red. In this case the nature of the supplying should be carefully considered. Heat is a *yang* form of energy and supplying with moxa will increase the imbalance by strengthening an already over-strong *yang* condition. The supplying should be with needles or other non-invasive techniques.

13

Musculo-skeletal problems

13.1 JOINT DISORDERS

13.1.1 Local non-arthritic joint disorders

Palpation of the superficial and deep structures is an important aspect of diagnosis. If there is superficial tenderness and heat, then according to TCM the tendino-muscular meridian (TM) would be considered over-active relative to the main meridian which lies deeper in the tissues. Similarly if there is tenderness on deep palpation and pain on joint movement then the TM is considered to be under-active relative to the main meridian.

To balance the local deep and superficial energies, it follows that treatment will involve 'sedating' the over-active meridian at the same time as the under-active meridian is 'supplied'.

The location of the area of pain should be looked at with a view to identify which meridian is in the vicinity. For example, if there is an excess in the TM of the stomach meridian, this could cause pain on superficial pressure over the antero-lateral aspect of the knee. Over-activity in the TM is accompanied by under-activity in the main meridian. Treatment therefore must include sedation of the TM and supplying of the stomach meridian, i.e. the *ah shi* (most tender point) should be needled superficially and ST 42 (*chongyang*) the *yuan* (source) point of the stomach 'supplied'.

The principles of treatment described above are relevant to local problems and can be a very useful way to treat acute trauma. NB The sedation of the TM could be effected by a simple ice-pack rather than using needles.

13.1.2 Arthritic joint disorders

Treating an arthritic joint problem is approached in a different way in TCM. Traditional Chinese medicine identifies through the

Five Element Correspondences that the controlling influence on bones and joints are the kidney/bladder organs. For example, if a patient presents with a painful knee and X-rays have shown changes in the joint consistent with an osteoarthritic condition, the fact that there may be kidney/bladder involvement must be borne in mind. There are some questions on general health which need to be asked, which will confirm the diagnosis.

1. Does the patient need to get up to void the bladder during the night? Normally one sleeps through the night or may rise once only. Any more frequent incidences should be considered as abnormal.
2. Does the patient feel worse in cold weather? The external influence of the Water element is cold.
3. What is the overall impression of the complexion? Is there a greyish-blue underlying pallor? (The colour of the Water element is blue/black).
4. Is there a particular time of day when the pain is worse? The significant times are between 15.00 and 19.00 hours when energy is at its greatest in the Water element. Alternatively, the opposite time could be significant, i.e. 3.00 to 7.00 hours. At this time energy is at is weakest in the kidney and bladder organs and there may be a block in the energy cycle as it passes through the other organs of the *zang/fu* system.

(a) Tongue

Observation of the tongue can confirm the diagnosis. Typically it will be pale and have toothmarks at the edges. This is caused by inadequate fluid control by the kidney and spleen.

(b) Pulses

The pulses can also be used. The nature of the balance between kidney *yin* and *yang* energy can be felt in the deep proximal pulse of the left (kidney pulse) and right wrist (pericardium pulse) respectively. In clinical practice the most likely underlying diagnosis of an arthritic knee is a kidney *yin xu* condition. The points to supply will be a choice of:

- BL 23 (*shenshu*) which is the *shu* point of the kidney organ.

- SP 6 (*sanjinjiao*). This is influential in balancing the *yin* and *yang* energy in the kidney.
- KI 3 (*taixi*) the *yuan*/source point of the KI.

13.1.3 BI syndromes

BI means obstruction of *qi* and blood. This is due to invasion of Wind, Damp and Cold, when the body is weak.

(a) Wandering BI

This describes the flitting pain from joint to joint in the extremities and indicates a predominance of Wind.

Tongue: thin yellow coat.
Pulses: superficial and rapid.
Acupoints: BL 17 (*geshu*), SP 10 (*xuehai*) plus local points.
Needling technique: superficial and reducing.

(b) Painful BI

Arthralgia which is relieved with heat and exacerbated by cold. This indicates a predominance of Cold.

Tongue: thin white coat.
Pulses: tight and wiry.
Acupoints: BL 23 (*shenshu*), CV 4 (*guanyuan*), plus local points.
Needling technique: deep, supplying plus moxa.

(c) Fixed BI

Numbness and heavines in the joints provoked by damp weather. This indicates a predominance of Damp.

Tongue: white sticky coat.
Pulses: slow.
Acupoints: ST 36 (*zusanli*), SP 6 (*sanyinjiao*) plus local points.
Technique: cupping, moxa, needling (supplying).

(d) Febrile BI

Arthralgia with local redness and hot swelling, in one or several joints. This indicates the Wind, Cold and Damp have turned to Heat.

Tongue: yellow dry coat.
Pulses: slippery and rapid.
Acupoints: GV 14 (*dazui*), LI 11 (*quchi*), plus local points.
Needling technique: reducing and superficial.

13.1.4 Differentiating between a *yin* and *yang* condition

The diagnosis can be confused if the joint presents hot and swollen. It is important to differentiate between a local *yang* condition and a systemic *yin* condition. The latter can be ascertained from the history and examination of the pulses and tongue. Treatment would then be formulated to reduce the *yang* condition locally but also to 'supply' the acupoints that will replenish KI *qi*.

13.2 MUSCLE DISORDERS

A great deal of time is spent in clinical practice, coping with painful conditions affecting the muscles and tendons. Diagnosis in Western terms will address the problem locally. A treatment programme will be worked out accordingly, which will aim to relieve pain and restore function.

TCM looks at the problem from a more systemic point of view. A disorder in the muscles is the result of a problem in the Wood element, the affected organs being the gall bladder/liver. The external climatic condition is Wind (*fong*).

Wind is believed to enter the body at GB 20 (*fenchi*). The location of this point on the outer third of the occiput puts it above normal collar height and therefore it is susceptible to invasion of Wind.

13.2.1 Superficial invasion of Wind

If the penetration is superficial it might give rise to pain and stiffness in the cervical spine. For example, a patient may wake in the morning with a stiff neck, having retired to bed perfectly fit and well. A traditional Chinese explanation would be, that perverse energy Wind and Cold has penetrated at GB 20 (*fenchi*) because the head and neck are exposed to draughts. The same criteria of examination and treatment apply as for the acute joint condition described above. The meridian involved will mainly be the gall bladder in this case.

If the Wind penetrates into the main gall bladder meridian a more systemic treatment must be considered. For example, the patient presents with a stiff painful shoulder. On examination, there is limitation of movement in all directions. X-ray examination shows no bony changes. Chinese diagnosis would describe this condition as a disruption of the smooth passage of *qi* through the shoulder, due to the invasion of Wind, Cold and Damp. This can be confirmed by:

1. Carefully ascertaining when the symptoms began; whether they were gradual/sudden in onset; whether they were preceded by any cervical pain or stiffness; whether there was trauma.
2. Finding out if the symptoms are worse between 23.00 and 3.00 hrs (Wood element time).

    Experience in clinical practice bears out the fact that shoulder pain is worse in bed at night. The patient may also experience an increase of pain during the day between 11.00 and 15.00 hrs when energy is at its lowest in the liver/gall bladder.
3. There are unlikely to be bladder continence problems, as with the painful knee example above. There may be, however, a feeling of fullness in the head which could manifest as a headache or irritability/impatience. Anger is the emotion of the Wood element and these symptoms would further confirm a disorder in liver/gall bladder.
4. Any exposure to draught or wind prior to the symptoms occurring or dislike of wind would further confirm a disturbance in Wood. (Wind is the external perverse influence of Wood.)

    In formulating a treatment programme local points used could be: GB 20 (*fengchi*), GB 21 (*jianjing*), eyes of shoulder; TE 14 (*jianliao*), LI 15 (*jianyu*). Distal points: GB 34 (*yanglinguan*) specific for muscle and tendon. LR 3 (*taichong*) *yuan* source point.

13.2.2 The aims of treatment

These will include the normal aims identified in Western practice plus aims relevant to the Chinese diagnosis.

A possible list of aims is:

1. To relieve pain.
2. To restore function.

3. To restore the balance of *qi* and to eliminate the invading pathogens, e.g. Wind, Cold, Damp.
4. To teach the patient how to maintain this balance of *qi* and restored function.

These aims can be met by standard physical treatment combined with acupuncture. The physical methods used to achieve the above aims will vary depending on the basic training of the practitioner but may include mobilizing/manipulation, facilitation techniques, electrotherapy, hot/cold therapy, exercise, postural correction, advice on lifestyle and diet.

Acupuncture can be added with two aims in mind.

1. As a technique using either invasive or non-invasive acupuncture for relief of pain.
2. To help restore the balance of *qi* in the *zang/fu* system.

Acupuncture treatment should be planned to include local treatment for relief of pain and systemic treatment to eliminate the identified pathogens. For example:

- LI 11 (*quchi*) is effective in eliminating Heat.
- ST 36 (*zusanli*) and SP 6 (*sanjinjiao*) are effective in eliminating Damp.
- BL 23 (*shenshu*) heated with moxa to eliminate Cold.
- BL 17 (*geshu*) is effective in eliminating Wind.

13.3 ACUPOINTS COMMONLY USED IN MUSCULO-SKELETAL CONDITIONS

Listed below are local and distal acupuncture points that are most effective in some musculo-skeletal conditions. The list gives a selection of local points and is not intended as a prescription for all complaints. It is up to the practitioner to identify the area affected and then select the points accordingly.

13.3.1 Cervical spine

Local: GB 20 (*fenchi*), 21 (*jianjing*), BL 10 (*tianzhu*), SI 14 (*jianwaishu*), SI 15 (*jianzhongshu*), TE 16 (*tianyou*), TE 17 (*yifeng*), GV 15 (*yamen*). Extra 21 (*huatuojiaji*).

Distal: GB 34 (*yanglinguan*), *ho* point and specific for tendon and muscle. GB 39 (*xuanshong*) for rigidity of cervical spine.

13.3.2 Thoracic spine

Local: points along the bladder and GV meridian. Extra 21 (*huatuojiaji*) (Figure 13.1).
Distal: BL 40 (*weizhong*).

13.3.3 Upper extremity (Figures 13.2 and 13.3)

(a) Shoulder

Local: The eyes of the shoulder, i.e. *chien chien* (1 inch above axilla crease anteriorly) and *chien hau* (1 inch above the axilla crease posteriorly), SI 10 (*naoshu*), LI 14 (*binao*), LI 15 (*jianyu*), LI 16 (*jugu*), TE 14 (*jianliao*).
Distal: *ho* points: LI 11 (*quchi*), TE 10 (*tianjing*).

When the shoulder is stiff: ST 38 (*tiaokou*) on the same side combined with GB 41 (foot *linqi*) on the opposite side. Move

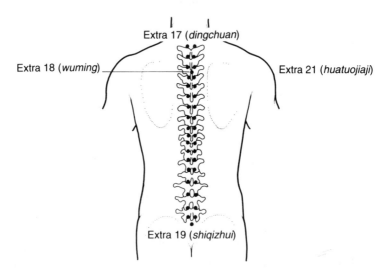

Figure 13.1 The acupuncture points Extra 21 (*huatuojiaji*), Extra 17 (*dingchuan*), Extra 18 (*wuming*) and Extra 19 (*shiqizui*).

the shoulder while these two needles are *in situ* to improve mobility.

(b) Elbow

Local: LI 11 (*quchi*), LI 12 (*zhouliao*), LU 5 (*chize*), HT 3 (*shaohai*), TE 10 (*tianjing*).

Distal: LI 4 (*hegu*), GB 34 (*yanglinguan*).

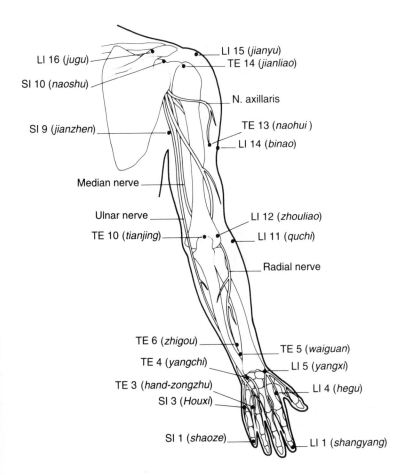

Figure 13.2 The relationship between the main points of the lateral aspect of the upper extremities and the nerves.

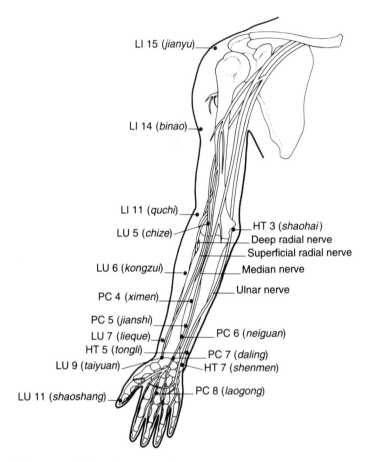

Figure 13.3 The relationship between the main points of the medial aspect of the upper extremities and the nerves.

(c) Wrist

Local: LI 5 (*yangxi*), LI 4 (*hegu*), TE 4 (*yangchi*), HT 7 (*shenmen*), LI 9 (taiyuan), PC 7 (*daling*), Extra 25 (*zhonquan*).
Distal: LI 11 (*quchi*).

(d) Fingers

Local: Extra points 28 *baxie* (Figure 13.4). Needle and then heat with Moxa for stiffness in the joints and relief of pain.

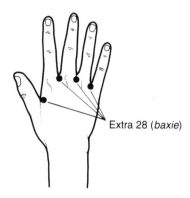

Extra 28 (*baxie*)

Figure 13.4 Acupoint Extra 28 (*baxie*).

13.3.4 Lumbar spine

Local: points on bladder line in particular BL 24 (*qihaishu*) which is the *shu* point for lumbar spine. Extra 21 (*huatuojiaji*), GV 3 (*yaoyangguan*), GV 4 (*mingmen*).
Distal: BI 40 (*weizhong*).

13.3.5 Sacral spine

Local: points on bladder line. Extra 19 (*shiqizhui*) located immediately below spinous process of 5th lumbar vertebra (Figure 13.1).
Distal: BL 40 (*weishong*).

13.3.6 Lower extremity (Figures 13.5 and 13.6)

(a) Hip

Local: GB 30 (*huantiao*), GB 29 (femur *juliao*). In cases of OA hip three points superior, anterior and posterior to the greater trochanter can be needled to 5 cm depth and heated with moxa (Figure 13.7).
Distal: GB 34 (*yanglinguan*).

(b) Knee

Local: Stomach 34 (*liangqui*), ST 35 (*dubi*) with Extra 32 (*xiyan*) and extra 31 (*heding*) (Figure 13.8), SP 9 (*yinlingquan*), LR 8

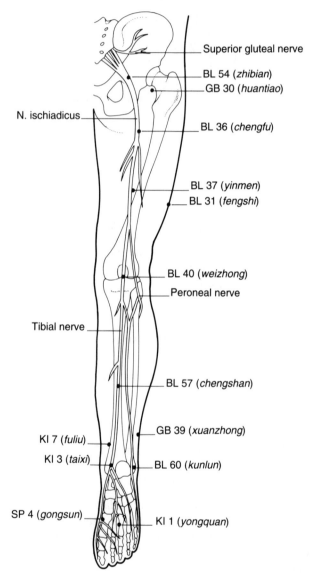

Figure 13.5 The relationship between the main points of the posterior aspect of the lower extremities and the nerves.

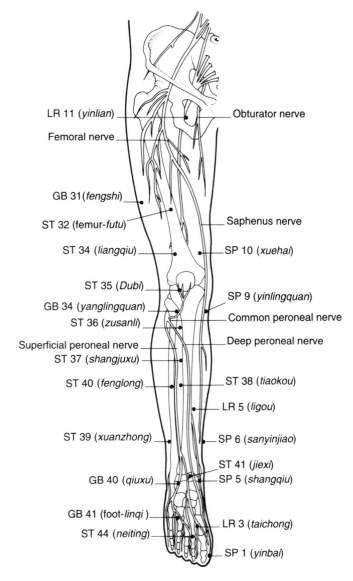

Figure 13.6 The relationship between the main points of the anterior aspect of the lower extremities and the nerves.

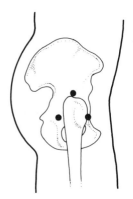

Figure 13.7 Extra points for osteoarthritis of the hip, to be treated with heated needles.

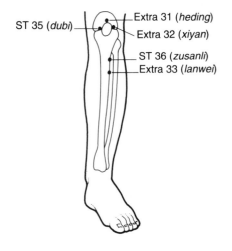

ST 35 (*dubi*) — Extra 31 (*heding*)
Extra 32 (*xiyan*)
ST 36 (*zusanli*)
Extra 33 (*lanwei*)

Figure 13.8 Extra points around the knee joint.

(*ququan*), BL 39 (*weiyang*) – this point can be needled and heated with moxa for chronic arthritis, BL 40 (*weizhong*).
Distal: ST 36 (*zusanli*), GB 34 (*yanglinguan*).

(c) Ankle

Local: ST 41 (*jiexi*), GB 40 (*qiuxu*), SP 5 (*shangqiu*), BL 60 (*kunlun*), BL 62 (*shenmai*), KI 3 (*taixi*).

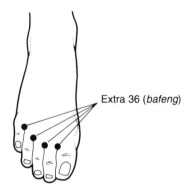

Extra 36 (*bafeng*)

Figure 13.9 Extra 36 (*bafeng*) points.

Distal: ST 36 (*zusanli*), GB 34 (*yanglinguan*), BL 40 (*weizhong*).

(d) Ist MTP joint

Local: SP 2 (*dadu*), SP 3 (*taibai*).
Distal: SP 9 (*yinlingquan*).

(e) Toes

Local: Extra 36 (*bafeng*) (Figure 13.9). Needle and heat with Moxa.

13.4 SYSTEMIC TREATMENT

There are some painful joint disorders that are in fact the result of autoimmune disease as in rheumatoid arthritis. In these cases a different approach to treatment is indicated. This is where the eight extra meridians can be used, e.g. SI 3 (*houxi*) plus BL 62 (*shenmai*). These are the key points of *du mai* and *yang wei mai*, which traditionally are believed to affect the autoimmune system. Use of these key points is looking to a long term-effect on the condition.

If the patient is on systemic cortisone this tends to block the effect of acupuncture initially and patients should be advised that the effect of acupuncture will not be felt immediately.

Advice on lifestyle should also be an important aspect of treatment. Close cooperation with other health professionals in the long-term management of progressive joint diseases is essential.

These include the occupational therapist for expertise in the aids to daily living, the social worker, district nurse and the general practitioner and consultant.

13.5 OTHER TECHNIQUES

13.5.1 Ear acupuncture

The appropriate area designated on the ear corresponding to the anatomical area being treated can be stimulated along with body points. This can be achieved by using simple needling, laser or electro-stimulation. Other points may be stimulated, i.e.

- Ear point *shenmen* for calming effect and relaxation.
- Kidney point for stimulating KI *qi*.
- Sympathetic point to augment pain relief.
- Liver/gall bladder point if problem is muscular.

13.5.2 Ear acupressure

A seed or wood chip can also be applied to the appropriate point(s) to give a constant stimulation between clinic attendances.

13.5.3 Trigger point acupuncture

This can be used for local muscular problems as well as designated acupoints to affect the body systemically. For example, local pain in the shoulder can be treated with trigger point acupuncture and GB 34 (*yanglinguan*) added as a point which influences muscles. While the local needles will be used in a superficial way as described in Chapter 10, the needle in GB 34 (*yanglinguan*) would be left *in situ* for 15–20 minutes to supply the point. This form of acupuncture can be very effective in short-term relief of pain. This may be all that is needed to break an established pain pattern when the underlying cause of the pain has been resolved.

It can also be used for pain relief prior to mobilizing. If however it is used prior to manipulating the anaesthetic effect should not be forgotten and the natural muscle protection will be inhibited.

Without this protection damage could be caused. Personal experience has demonstrated a good result from using this technique prior to assisted joint movement and Maitland mobilizing techniques to grade III level only.

13.5.4 Transcutaneous electrical nerve stimulation

This can be applied over acupoints and then left with the patient to use at home between treatments. Alternatively it can be applied between sessions when needles are used, in order to continue stimulating the acupoints between treatments.

13.6 CASE STUDIES

13.6.1 Tennis elbow

Mrs Z., age 49, secretary, likes playing tennis.

History

Ten-month history of right tennis elbow. She had had two injections of hydrocortisone and had been to an osteopath several times.

On examination

There was local tenderness over the common extensor origin (CEO). Extension was reduced by 10%.

Cervical spine: Prominence of C7 with head held forward with increase of lordosis. Full range of movement but pain was felt on overpressure on right rotation. Tenderness locally of the C2–T2 apophyseal joints (right).

Assessment

This was a combined problem involving the cervical spine and elbow. Aim of treatment:

1. To relieve pain in elbow.
2. To correct neck posture.
3. To analyse working posture and improve if necessary.

Treatment

Acupuncture locally using *ah shi* (local tender point), LI 11 (*quchi*), distal point LI 4 (*hegu*). Discussion of sitting posture and periodic cervical correction while working.
Second treatment one week later. There was no improvement. Treatment: Maitland mobilization using postero-anterior techniques to the apophyseal joints C2–T2. Repeat of local acupuncture. GB 34 (*yanglinguan*) was added as a distal point and for its specific effect on muscles and tendons.
Third treatment one week later. Some improvement. Tenderness less marked and patient now had full extension of right elbow. Neck movement was full and pain-free. Repeat of acupuncture and discussion of working posture plus advice on padding tennis racket handle. This puts less strain on the common extensor tendon when gripping the handle.
Fourth treatment one week later. Further improved but still some local tenderness. Repeat of acupuncture using the same points. Patient advised to return if relapsed or if no further improvement. Working on the principle that the three factors identified had been addressed the in-built body healing would complete the job.

13.6.2 Knee joint

Mrs H., hairdresser, age 55.

History

Several years increasing stiffness and pain in right knee. Diagnosed as osteoarthritis. Conventional physiotherapy had been of only temporary benefit. She admitted that she was not doing the recommended exercises advised during her last course of treatment. She had had bilateral stripping of veins in the legs and four weeks previously an arthroscopy of the right knee. This had shown advanced joint changes and the surgeon had suggested a total knee replacement as the only avenue left.

On examination

There was full range of movement in both knees but pain at both mid range and at full flexion in the right knee. There was some difficulty in doing static quadriceps contraction bilaterally.

Assessment

There was no significant organ imbalance demonstrated and local treatment was decided on initially.

Aim of treatment:

1. To relieve pain.
2. To improve the strength of the muscles controlling the knee.

Treatment

Acupuncture to BL 39 (*weiyang*) heated with Moxa. Local points: ST 35 (*dubi*), local point medial side patella tendon. Quadriceps drill.

Second treatment one week later. Very much better. Still some pain felt on climbing up and down stairs. Treatment repeated as before. Patient then went away to the country for a holiday. On her return she was able to report that she had been able to go on long walks without ill effect and that the pain was now minimal going up and down stairs. Continuation of the home programme of exercises was emphasized and the patient discharged.

13.6.3 Shoulder A

Mr S., age 62.

History

Pain for eight months following a 'missed smash' while playing badmintion. Now not so severe, but does wake twice during the night with the pain.

On examination

Shoulder movement: Elevation, extension and abduction full with pain at end of range. Medial rotation was two-thirds of normal range and lateral rotation was three-quarters of normal range. All movement was painful.

Cervical spine: All movements were slightly restricted and the facet joint of C5 right was very tender to palpation.

Assessment

This was a condition caused by pathogenic invasion of Wind.

Treatment

GB 20 (*fengchi*), 21 (*jiangjing*) (right), 'Eyes' of shoulder LI 4 (*hegu*). Maitland postero-anterior grade II right C5 facet joint.

Second treatment: one week later. Sleeping well, pain less severe. Treatment was repeated on two further occasions and the patient discharged clear of pain and with full range of movement in the shoulder and cervical spine.

13.6.4 Shoulder B

Mrs C., age 43.

History

Nine years of pain in the right shoulder. She sits at a computer all day and also has a tennis elbow (right). She had had a course of physiotherapy treatment consisting of heat and exercise, had been fitted with a cervical collar and epycondylitis cuff for her tennis elbow symptoms.

On examination

(a) Elbow. There was some wasting of the extensor muscles of the forearm and reduced grip.
(b) Shoulder. There was normal range of movement with pain on abduction and medial rotation at end of range.
(c) Cervical spine. Posture was very poor. A dorsal kyphosis with prominent C7 spinous process and increased cervical lordosis. The posture was only partially correctable. There was reduction of movement in all directions but there was no pain on movement. There was no yielding on manual overpressure at the end of range.

Assessment

This was primarily a postural problem giving rise to pain. Aim of Treatment:

1. To relieve pain.
2. To improve posture.

Treatment

GB 20, 21, 34: These are local and distal points on the GB channel. LI 11 local point. TH 5 local point for arm pain.

Shown neck bracing exercise to practise against pillow before sleeping and on waking.

Second treatment one week later. There had been two pain-free days but now all the symptoms had returned. On examination there was increase in range of extension in the cervical spine. Treatment was repeated as before.

Third treatment one week later. Now much better. Less pain in shoulder but still weakness and discomfort in the forearm. Repeat treatment.

Fourth treatment. Two weeks later. No pain now in shoulder and movement was full and pain-free. The forearm symptoms were much improved. The patient was discharged having had the postural advice reinforced.

13.7 CONCLUSIONS

Treatment of musculo-skeletal problems using a combination of Western and traditional Chinese diagnosis and techniques can be very rewarding.

An understanding of systemic *xu* or *shih* conditions is important to improve the effectiveness of treatment. Advice on exercise, posture and lifestyle all form an essential part of a rehabilitation programme.

14

Respiratory disorders

Acupuncture has a great deal to offer in respiratory disorders. As yet there is not the body of research data available in the West to validate the effects of acupuncture on respiratory disorders. This is slowly being rectified (Jobst *et al.*, 1986 and Fung *et al.*, 1986). Personal experience in this area has proved very rewarding.

14.1 THE FUNCTION OF THE LUNG ORGAN

In TCM the lung has the vital function of using the *t'ai qi* from fresh air and converting it to *zong qi* which is then dispersed throughout the body. It also controls the skin and temperature regulation through the sweat glands and body hair. It has important functional links with the large intestine, spleen and kidney.

14.1.1 LI and LU

Qi is sent down to the LI which is its paired *fu* organ, to enable the fuctional separation of impure and pure fluids to be completed and the bowels to function smoothly.

If there is insufficient *qi* descending to the LI there is reduced activity and bowel movement resulting in constipation. The clear passage of descending *qi* is blocked and the result is distension in the chest and bronchial asthma.

14.1.2 Lung and spleen

Qi is sent down to the spleen to enable it to function as a transporter and transformer of food and drink. This then sends nourishment to the LU.

If *qi* is weak in the SP, the spleen function is impaired. This leads to insufficient nourishment to the LU and reduced LU *qi*. This can be manifested in two ways.

1. Insufficiency of *qi* causes lassitude, loose stools, shortness of breath and a disinclination to talk. This then leads to:
2. Accumulation of body fluids in the interior (Damp-Phlegm), asthma, cough, and excessive sputum.

14.1.3 Lung and kidney

The kidney is the store of *yuan qi* (ancestral energy) which is used by the lung to convert the *t'ai qi* inspired from fresh air to *zong qi*, which is then dispersed to facilitate all the functions of the *zang/fu*. The *yin qi* of these two organs nourish each other and they are interdependent. Impairment of kidney function leads to reduced lung function. This can lead to inspiration dyspnoea, severe cough, asthma and oedema.

RESPIRATORY DISORDERS MET IN CLINICAL PRACTICE

14.2 ASTHMA

A Western concept of asthma is that of constriction of the bronchioles which can be brought about by a variety of causes, which include allergy, infection and emotional upset.

The TCM concept looks at the lungs as the organ reponsible for the tranformation and distribution of *qi* and regards asthma as a series of symptoms associated with a variety of perverse influences on lung function. Thus three types of asthma are identified: *shi* type, *xu* type, mixed type.

14.2.1 *Shi* type

This can be caused by:

(a) invasion of Wind-Cold;
(b) accumulation of Damp-Phlegm.

(a) Invasion of Wind-Cold

This inhibits the LU in enabling the *qi* to descend and the symptoms include cough with thin sputum, shortness of breath, nasal congestion, and runny nose. Tongue: thin white coating. Pulse: superficial.

Treatment

- BL 13 (*feishu*), *shu* point of the LU;
- LU 7 (*lieque*), the *lo* point of the LU;
- LU 5 (*chize*), to pacify ascending *qi* and disperse the LU;
- LI 4 (*hegu*), to dispel Wind.

(b) Accumulation of Damp-Phlegm

This results from an inital invasion of Cold. Insufficiency of spleen *yang* leads to retention of cold fluid forming phlegm. This reduces the spleen function in its nourishment of the LU. The resulting symptoms include: rapid coarse breathing, stifling sensation in the chest, thick purulent sputum. Tongue: thick yellowish coating. Pulse: rapid and forceful.

Treatment

- LU 5 (*chize*) to cool heat;
- ST 40 (*fenglong*) to eliminate Damp;
- CV 22 (*tiantu*) to calm asthma, clear LU and resolve phlegm.
- Extra (*ding chuan*) to subdue ascending *qi*.

14.2.2 *Xu* type

This is due to the lung not receiving the necessary *yuan qi* to carry out its function of transforming *t'ai qi* from the air. This type of condition is a result of prolonged illness with chronic cough and is most likely to occur later in life. This can either be the result of lung *xu* or KI *xu*.

(a) Lung xu

Symptoms will include: short and rapid breathing, weak and low voice, weak cough with thin sputum. The patient will be tired and have a pale complexion. Tongue: pale, toothmarked. Pulse: weak.

Treatment

- BL 13 (*feishu*) *shu* point of the lung;
- BL 43 (*gaohuangshu*) to tonify *yuan qi* (NB this point is 3 *cun* lateral to the lower border of the 4th thoracic vertebra);

- LU 9 (*taiyuan*) the *yuan* point of the LU meridian;
- ST 36 (*zusanli*) to tonify SP and ST and stimulate *qi* to whole meridian system.

(b) Kidney xu

The symptoms include: dyspnoea on exertion, asthma, chilliness with cold extremities, difficulty breathing in. Tongue: pale and wet. Pulse: deep, thready and weak.

14.2.3 Mixed type

There are many ways in which the different pathogens can combine to cause asthma. Here are some of the most common combinations met in clinical practice.

(a) LU xu and invasion of Wind-Cold

This is frequently seen in children but also in adults. The LU *xu* leads to *wei qi xu* which means that the patient easily catches cold.

Treatment
In an acute attack the treatment is designed to get rid of Wind-Cold and in between attacks the *xu* condition should be corrected and *qi* strengthened. In China children are treated every month during the summer in order to minimize attacks of asthma during the winter.

(b) LU xu and Damp-Phlegm or Heat-Phlegm

Frequently seen in adults and is often the result of overwork and improper diet. Too many fatty foods contribute to internal damp-phlegm.

Treatment
This is aimed at tonifying LU and SP *qi* using back *shu* points and dispersing phlegm using channel points. For example:

- BL 20 (*pishu*) *shu* point of the spleen;
- BL 13 (*feishu*) *shu* point of the lung;
- LU 9 (*taiyuan*) *yuan* point of LU and to dispel phlegm;
- SP 6 (*sanyinjiao*) to eliminate Damp and strengthen SP *xi*;

- ST 40 (*fenglong*) to dispel heat-phlegm and damp-phlegm;
- CV 17 (*shanzhong*) to regulate *qi* and subdue ascending *qi*, to clear the lung and resolve phlegm.

(c) LU xu, heat-phlegm and KI xu

This has similar results to type (b) but is suffered by a more elderly age group particularly after long chronic illness. In this case the KI *xu* condition needs to be addressed. The following points can be added:

- BL 23 (*shenshu*) *shu* point of KI;
- CV 4 (*guanyan*) to tonify KI and strengthen *yang qi*;
- CV 6 (*qihai*) to tonify the kidney;
- GV 4 (*mingmen*) to strengthen the KI and tonify *yuan qi*.

14.2.4 Use of Moxa

This can be used to 'supply' on BL 13 (*feishu*) and Extra 17 (*dingchuan*) (Figure 13.1) if there is a *xu* condition. As a first aid measure, patients can be advised to put a hot water bottle over the upper thoracic spine when breathing is distressed and also shown how to use acupressure on LU 7 (*lieque*) and CV 17 (*shanzhong*).

14.2.5 Ear points for asthma

These can be stimulated by laser, electro-stimulation or acupressure. The points most used are:

- ear point *shenmen* for sedating effect;
- lung point: organ point;
- *dingchuan*: specific for asthma.

If a patient is on steroid treatment acupuncture is less effective. One of the benefits of acupuncture treatment is that the dose of steroid can be reduced. This must only be attempted in cooperation with the patient's medical practitioner.

14.3 HAY FEVER

This is a condition which is interesting in that it can affect some people while others remain unaffected, the lifestyle of both groups being similar. Skin irritation is often associated with this problem. It is usually seasonal, hence its name. Some manifest symptoms early in the spring, others later and yet others have symptoms throughout the year. It would appear that different people are vulnerable to different external pathogenic influences.

The symptoms can be looked at and analysed in a similar way to that described in differentiating different forms of asthma. The internal pathogens should not be ignored and correction of diet can prove rewarding in long-term alleviation of this condition.

The symptoms presented are of sneezing, running nose, red eyes and shortness of breath. These symptoms suggest invasion of Wind, rising liver *yang* and Damp-Phlegm.

There are a series of points described in the Chinese texts which have a particular effect on allergy:

- SP 10 (*xuehai*) specific for allergy. Used particularly to cool the blood, as in urticaria for example. NB the spleen is mother to lung.
- GV 20 (*baihui*) the meeting point of all the *yang* meridians and a sedating point.
- LI 4 (*hegu*), dispels Wind.
- LI 11 (*quchi*), reduce heat.
- LI 20 (*yingxiang*), local to the nose.
- Extra 1 (*yintang*) (Figure 14.1). This should be needled horizontally downwards.
- LU 7 (*lieque*) *lo* point and to promote the dispersal function of lung.
- BL 13 (*feishu*) *shu* point of lung.
- LR 3 (*taichong*) (to calm rising *yang qi* and dispel Wind).

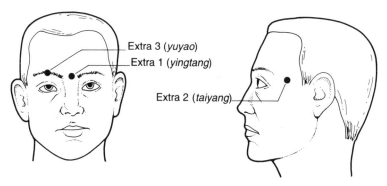

Figure 14.1 Extra points on the forehead.

14.4 BRONCHITIS

This is a chronic condition of the lungs. It is exacerbated by seasonal changes in the weather, polluted air and cigarette smoke. Treatment of this condition is based on the principles of Chinese diagnosis described above.

14.4.1 Some useful acupoints in chronic cases

- BL 13 (*feishu*) *shu* point of lung;
- LU 1 (*zhongfu*) *mu* point of lung;
- LU 7 (*lieque*) and KI 6 (*zhaohai*) the key points of *ren mai* and *yin chiao mai*;
- BL 20 (*pishu*) for excessive sputum;
- CV 12 (*zhongwan*) for abdominal distension.

14.4.2 Useful points in acute attacks

Select points along the lung channel:

- LU 5 (*chize*) *ho* point of LU;
- LU 7 (*lieque*) *luo* point of LU;
- LI 4 (*hegu*) *yuan* point of LI;
- ST 40 (*fenglong*) for excessive sputum.

14.4.3 Points to improve *qi* to resist infection

- ST 36 (*zusanli*)
- CV 6 (*qihai*)
- GV 14 (*dazhui*)

14.4.4 Treatment for nicotine withdrawal symptoms

Nicotine addiction is believed to be one of the most difficult to overcome. If a patient with bronchitis or bronchial asthma wants to give up smoking this should be considered an important aspect of the treatment programme.

Ear points can be successfully utilized in nicotine addiction. The points lung and *shenmen* are effective. These can be augmented by general body acupuncture aimed at replenishing *qi* and also soothing agitation.

LI 4 (*hegu*) moves *qi*.
LR 3 (*taichong*) draws energy down.
ST 36 (*zusanli*) replenishes *qi* in the meridian system.

14.5 POST-OPERATIVE CHEST PROBLEMS

One of the major tasks in physiotherapy is that of preventing post-operative chest complications following general anaesthetic. In most cases there is no complication but some patients, especially those who smoke, do get excessive secretions and patients with abdominal wounds are reluctant to cough because of the severe pain caused.

Personal experience has demonstrated an effective way of getting a productive cough in these cases. Acupressure on CV 17 (*shanzhong*) and on BL 13 (*feishu*) facilitates the cough and reduces the effort that has to be made in expectoration. Patients can be shown how to stimulate CV 17 for themselves and then combine this with a 'huffing' technique to produce sputum. ST 40 (*fenglong*) can also be treated in this way.

14.6 CASE STUDIES

14.6.1 Hay fever

Mr L., age 60, had had hay fever for 20 years. The symptoms at the height of the season were severe enough to curtail normal working or socializing. He had come for treatment following a *Which* article recommending acupuncture as a hay fever cure.

On examination, there was nothing significant in either pulses or tongue. He was feeling reasonably well but there was some irritation of the eyes and increase of nasal mucus.

Treatment

I used a simple formula as described in the traditional Chinese texts: LI 4, 11, 20, plus *ying tang*, an extra point between the eyebrows (Figure 13.10) and LR 3 (*taichong*) to bring energy down from the head. All needles were retained for 20 minutes and stimulated manually once during that period.

Second treatment: There was no further development of symptoms after 10 days. Treatment was repeated as above adding GV 20, a specific point calming *yang* symptoms.

He was treated at weekly intervals during which time he had some symptoms but these were very much reduced compared to other years. The pollen count was very high during that period. After four treatments he was clear of symptoms. A further three treatments were given and the patient discharged.

The following year he came again prior to the hay fever season and had three treatments at weekly intervals using the points described above. This man has had no further recurrence of hay fever in 6 years.

It is interesting to note that in the same year of his first course of treatment, in October, he developed severe urticaria and had to be admitted to hospital and given cortisone treatment. In traditional Chinese medicine there is an association between the lungs and the skin through the Metal element. I did not immediately make this connection until I heard Dr Jayasuriya from the World Health Organization Hospital in Colombo, talking about his own experience of treating long-standing conditions too quickly. He described a young man with a long-standing gravitational ulcer on the ankle which he had resolved with acupuncture treatment within four weeks. The young man returned soon after with asthmatic symptoms which he had never experienced previously.

I consider that my patient was treated too severely with acupuncture earlier in the year. There was a long-standing imbalance in the Metal element which I did not take fully into account. The symptoms of the hay fever which are basically respiratory were too quickly treated and the urticaria was the reaction of the overstressed Metal element in the autumn. It was a sobering lesson to be more careful in treating long-standing problems too quickly.

With hindsight, the use of a formula without taking into account other factors of the *sheng* cycle is not to be recommended. I have, however, used the LI acupoints described above in many other cases with success, but have combined them with other acupoints appropriate to the individual patient. I recommend treatment at weekly intervals four weeks before the hay fever season commences and attendance to control actual symptoms is usually necessary only once or twice during the height of the season.

14.7 CONCLUSIONS

It is very worthwhile to consider using acupuncture in respiratory conditions. It should be remembered that disorders affecting the skin can also be treated using the principles described for respiratory conditions, as skin is influenced by the lung and colon.

When treating a long-standing disorder it is better to have a slow steady improvement rather than a rapid correction, as this could lead to further problems.

A close relationship with the patient's medical practitioner is essential in order that medication can be adjusted as the condition changes.

REFERENCES

Jobst, K., McPherson, K., Brown, V., Fletcher, H., Mole, P., Jin Hua Chen, Efthimiou, J., Maciocia, G., Shifron, K., and Lane, D. (1986) Controlled trial of acupuncture for disabling breathlessness. *Lancet*, Dec 20/27th.

Kam Pui Fung, Olivia Kit Wun Chow, and Shun Yeung So (1986) Attenuation of exercise induced asthma by acupuncture. *Lancet*, Dec 20/27th.

15

Pain

Pain is probably the most common condition that is faced in clinical practice.

In TCM pain may be classified as *xu* (deficient) or *shi* (excess). *Shi* generally represents the most painful conditions and is the result of either stagnation of *qi* and blood or cold, the latter giving rise to the most severe pain, whereas *xu* is caused by insufficient nourishment of *qi* and blood which results in reduced circulation of *qi* through the *zang fu* system.

If *qi* flows freely through the organs and meridian system the normal functions of the body can continue without restriction. If there is a block to this flow of *qi* these functions are inhibited and this gives rise, in most cases, to a degree of pain. Finding the underlying fault in the circulation of *qi* is a problem-solving exercise which brings into play the examination and diagnostic techniques addressed in Part One.

At the same time the basic knowledge of the physiology of pain can be brought into play. Electrical stimulation of chosen acupoints designed to facilitate the movement of *qi* through the meridian system can also be stimulated at different frequencies to initiate the short and long-term responses to pain relief by the spinal cord and brain. The effect of insertion of needles into points local to the pain without electrical stimulation will also stimulate the mechanisms to give local short-term relief, while the distal points will stimulate the mechanisms giving long-term relief.

Short-term relief of pain using acupuncture can enable painful joints to be mobilized and/or exercised and be incorporated in a full rehabilitation programme. Immediate relief of pain is important, but should the examination indicate an underlying imbalance in the deeper energic areas this also has to be addressed.

In all treatment programmes the practitioner should logically work out what effect is required and use the knowledge of TCM and Western medicine accordingly.

15.2 CASE STUDIES

15.2.1 Hip and lumbar pain

History

Miss B., age 21, complained of pain in the right groin and at anterior superior iliac spine (ASIS), which was worse after swimming and aerobics. No particular cause was discovered. Local ultrasound had not helped and she was controlling the discomfort with co-proximal when necessary. There was a further complication, in that she was waiting to be admitted for a cholecystectomy.

On examination

There was full range of movement in the right hip with pain at the limit of internal and external rotation. There was full range movement in the lumbar spine and no apparent joint problem when palpated but there was local tenderness on the ASIS. In prone lying there was pain in the quadriceps muscle when the knee was fully flexed.

Assessment

My assessment was that this was a strain at the attachment of rectus femoris leading to incoordination of muscles acting on the hip, resulting in pain, although there might be referral of pain from the lumbar region as well.

Treatment

First treatment. Acupuncture: Local *ah shi* on origin of rectus femoris which lies close to the stomach channel and ST 36 (*zusanli*) as a distal point on the stomach channel.

Second treatment: No better. She was also in some distress with pain and nausea due to her gall bladder problem. On examination she still had a marked degree of tenderness in the area of the anterior superior iliac spine.

The same points were treated and GB 34 (*yanglingquan*) added, the latter point having a strong effect on the gall bladder and is also influential on muscles and tendons. The nausea subsided during the treatment.

Third treatment: there was no tenderness on palpating the origin of rectus femorus. The groin pain, however, was unchanged. The nausea was less severe. I decided to change the treatment to trigger-point acupuncture, bearing in mind the original assessment that pain could also be due to referred symptoms from the lumbar spine. Trigger points were located in erector spinae in the lumbar region and latissimus dorsi. This cleared the groin pain.

The patient was advised to ensure she fully stretched the quadriceps daily by lying prone and flexing the knee fully.

15.2.2 Stomach pain

Mrs C., age 40, complaining of discomfort in stomach area. Patient referred from medical registrar who had been unable to diagnose the cause of discomfort.

History

For two years increasing pain over the upper abdomen which was exacerbated when doing housework. There was also indigestion with fullness in the stomach after eating. She woke with pain about 7.00 am and it was at its most intense until 9.00 am (stomach time).

On examination

Area of skin of upper abdomen was hypersensitive. Deep pressure relieved tenderness. The tongue was pale with a red tip and toothmarks on either margin. It had a scant white fur.

It was interesting to note that the lady was born in mid-September and the time of day in which she felt the most pain was in the stomach time (Chapter 2).

The pulses indicated that the Earth was in excess and the Metal deficient.

Assessment

These findings led to the conclusion that there was a block in the stomach channel giving rise to congested *qi*. There were several ways to tackle the problem. Diet was inquired into, but nothing significant was elicited. It was decided to use local and distal points on the stomach meridian. An alternative treatment could have been to use Earth point on the LI 11 (*quchi*) to draw energy from the ST to the LI.

Treatment

First treatment: ST 23 (*taiyi*) bilateral. This point is significant for gastralgia and is local to the area of tenderness. ST 36 (*zusanli*). This is the *ho* point and used as a distal point. CV12 (*zhongwan*), also significant for gastralgia. Needles were retained for 15 minutes.

Second treatment: one week later. There was definite improvement in symptoms. The treatment was repeated.

Third treatment: one week later. Patient had good relief of pain but was still getting indigestion. A change of treatment was indicated as the symptom of indigestion had not changed although the abdominal pain was better. LI 4 (*hegu*) + LR 3 (*taichong*): these are used together to promote relaxation and to dissipate *yang*; CV 12 (*zhongwan*); ST 36 (*zusanli*); LI 11 (*quchi*): this is the Earth point of the LI.

Fourth treatment: one week later. Patient reported almost complete relief of symptoms. Treatment was repeated.

Fifth treatment: two weeks later. Improvement maintained on the whole but occasional feelings of emptiness in the stomach prior to eating. The tongue showed some yellow fur covering the central area. This indicated that there was some spleen dysfunction and SP 6 (*sanyinjiao*) was added to the other points.

Sixth treatment: two weeks later. Empty feeling before meals less than before but not entirely better. The yellow fur on the tongue was less thick. Patient felt more energetic and better in herself.

Seventh treatment: two weeks later. Still occasional indigestion but the pain had not returned. However, there was hypersensitivity over the upper abdomen. Trigger point acupuncture was used on the rectus abdominis, which gave immediate relief. ST 36 (*zusanli*). No further appointment was made.

15.2.3 Low abdominal pain

Mrs H., age 75. This lady was referred to me from a physiotherapist.

History

She complained of acute low abdominal pain which my colleague had recognized was not a musculo-skeletal problem. All investigations were negative, all treatment so far had failed to give relief. She was generally tired and was unable to do her usual housework, etc.

On examination

She was tender to deep palpation over the right groin. Her tongue was uncoated and unnaturally bright red. The pulses were all deep and *yin*. The water pulses were hardly palpable.

Assessment

This was a *yin* condition but had presented as a *yang* condition, i.e. the *yang* was overpowering *yin*.

The aims of treatment were:

1. To facilitate the free flow of *qi* away from the congested low abdominal area.
2. To restore the balance of *yin* and *yang qi*.

Treatment

First treatment: Local point to pain ST 29 (*guilai*), distal point ST 36 (*zusanli*) *ho* point; KI 3 (*taixi*) the *yuan*/source point. This point stimulates the *yin* energy in the kidney which is the source of *yuan qi* to the *zang/fu* system. The points were needled using a 'supplying' technique, i.e. the needles were left *in situ* for 20 minutes after achieving *deqi*.

Second treatment: one week later. Pain was less but still came in spasms although not so frequently. The tongue appeared marginally less bright and the pulses showed a definite improvement. The Water pulses were now palpable. The treatment was repeated.

Third treatment: one week later. The patient had been pain free for two days following treatment. Now some minimal discomfort. The tongue had returned to a normal healthy colour. This lady was discharged pain free after two more treatments.

15.2.4 Temporo-mandibular joint pain

Mrs W., age 54, severe temporo-mandibular joint (TMJ) pain.

History

Four months of pain, sudden onset, with no notable preceding incident to explain onset of pain. She had a long-standing history of rheumatoid arthritis. Medical treatment included a local injection of hydrocortisone into the TMJ with no lasting effect. On arrival at the physiotherapy department, she was in severe pain having refrained from taking any pain killers since early in the morning.

On initial examination

She was able to open her mouth only to one finger width. There appeared to be no limitation of cervical movement or tenderness of the upper cervical spine. (Many TMJ problems have a contributory factor of some joint involvement at C1 and C2 levels.)

Assessment

This was a pain caused by stuck *qi*. There was a choice of using local and distal points on the stomach channel ST 7 (*xiaguan*) and ST 36 (*zusanli*) or local and a distal point which is particularly effective for facial pain, i.e. LI 4 (*hegu*).

Treatment

There was an immediate need to relieve pain and TENS was applied: one electrode over ST 7 (*xianguan*, local to pain) and one electrode over LI 4 (*hegu*), which is the distal point used in facial pain. A simple continuous stimulation at approximately 80 Hz was applied. It is not possible to be precise when using some TENS machines. This particular model has two adjustments, intensity and frequency, both marked from 1 to 10, the lowest frequency being 15 Hz and the highest 100 Hz.

After 15 minutes the pain was relieved. The patient was then shown how to apply the treatment herself and sent away with her own machine and reviewed 3 days later. She was instructed to use the TENS stimulation for only one hour continuously and then to turn off the machine for three hours.

Second treatment: There had been marked relief of pain which had tempted her to stop using the TENS for 24 hours. During that period the pain had returned but with less intensity. She had an additional pain in the left maxilla which she felt was probably toothache.

On further examination

She was able to open her mouth to 2 finger widths. The area over the right TMJ was still very tender.

Treatment

Needles were used on this occasion: LI 4 (*hegu*) right and left (the latter for toothache in the left maxilla) ST 36 (*zusanli*) right, distal point of stomach meridian. An attempt was made to insert a needle at ST 7 (local to the TMJ) but the area was too tender. The needle was inserted superficially and removed straight away. The three remaining needles were left for 20 minutes, at the end of which time the toothache was clear and there was no further TMJ pain.

Third treatment: TMJ pain was completely relieved and she had been able to go to the dentist to have her tooth filled. She was not able to open her mouth fully but was happy to have the increased range of movement. She was discharged.

15.2.5 Groin/abdominal pain

Mrs D., age 54, complained of acute pain in right groin combined with flatulence and distension of the abdomen. Past medical history: cholecystectomy, 16 years previously.

History

Sudden onset of pain six months ago. The nature of the pain was deep and sharp, centred on the right pubic ramus. Bowel movement became erratic, alternating constipation and violent motions. Pain worse towards the end of the day and sometimes disturbed sleep. Extension of the hip relieved pain. Flexion increased pain. There had been some fear of malignant disease and full investigations had been carried out. All of these were negative.

On examination

The pulses were deep and *yin*, the tongue broad and pale pink with a thin white coating. Point of extreme tenderness near the location of ST 30. Corresponding tender point located in the right ear.

Assessment
This was a problem of the Middle Energizer, which involved the impairment of function of the stomach and spleen due to internal pathogenic Damp.

Treatment

ST 30 (*qichong*), 36 (*zusanli*): tender associated point in ear. The ear point was located using a point finder coupled to the needle inserted in ST 30. A small wooden chip was secured with micropore tape over the point located in the ear to be retained until the next visit. The nature of the pain and the bowel symptoms could have been contibuted to by some irritant food in the diet. It was suggested that she abstain from milk and added sugar in her diet. These are two of the most common foods that can contribute to internal pathogenic Damp causing erratic bowel symptoms.

Second treatment: One week later, she returned to report relief of pain for two days with some intermittent return of symptoms. On examination, pulses were less *yin*, the tongue unchanged.

Third treatment: Two weeks later the patient returned having had some days completely pain free but others with some pain. There was improvement in the bowel movements but they were still erratic.

Further treatment

LI 4 (*hegu*), ST 36 (*zusanli*), ST 30 (*qichong*). The choice of LI 4 (*hegu*) was for two reasons. It is a major point for pain and it is also an influential point in the LI meridian and could have some effect on the erratic bowel motions. Following this treatment the patient phoned to say that she was almost free of pain and that her bowels were now normal. She decided to continue with the simple exclusion diet.

15.2.6 Spinal pain

Ms D., age 30: This lady was admitted for intensive rehabilitation and was having difficulty in doing a comprehensive exercise programme because of severe pain.

History

Four years previously she had sustained an incomplete spinal cord injury at C2 level. She had complained of pain in her neck and shoulder, mainly on the right. She had never been without the pain since her injury. She described two sites of pain:

1. Right side of cervical spine and supra-spinatus area of the scapula.
2. Upper lumbar spine.

On initial examination

Cervical movement was restricted on right rotation. Other movements were normal. The two areas were very sensitive to touch and any light pressure induced severe pain locally.

Assessment

This was a case of unresolved pain due to spinal cord injury. There were two possible ways to deal with this patient.

1. Use local and distal points on the bladder and gall bladder meridians
2. Trigger point acupuncture. Palpation had elicited areas of acute tenderness associated with nodules in the muscles, namely upper fibres of trapezius, supra-spinatus and erector spinae.

Treatment

Trigger point acupuncture was used.

First treatment: the needles were left *in situ* for a maximum of only 30 seconds before the area was anaesthetized. Following this first treatment, the patient was free of pain and felt as if 'a weight had been lifted off her shoulders'.

Second treatment: the following day. There had been relief of pain for four hours but it had returned with full force and she had not slept well.

Assessment – too much was achieved too quickly. Although the needles had been carefully checked the swiftness of the anaesthetic effect probably meant that they had been retained too long.

Treatment – local trigger points as on the previous day but checking every 10 seconds. Deep needling to BL 24 (*qihaishu*) which is an influential point for lumbar spine; GV 4 (*mingmen*). There was relief of pain following treatment but not complete relief as on the previous day.

Third treatment: 5 days later. The patient had slept very well every night since the last treatment. All pain had gone from the cervical and shoulder area and there was a dull pain only, felt over the mid and upper lumbar spine.

On further examination

There was minimal tenderness on light palpation whereas there had been hypersensitivity in the same area at the start of the course of treatment.

Treatment

BL 23 (*shenshu*), the associated effect (*shu*) point of the kidney. BL 24 (*qihaishu*), influential point for lumbar pain. Following this treatment the pain did not return and the acupuncture was stopped. The patient was able to make the most of her remaining time in the rehabilitation programme.

15.2.7 Pain following spinal cord lesion

Mr S., age 25: The man was referred having been re-admitted to the spinal unit following a fall, in which he had sustained a fractured left tibia.

History

He had sustained a complete spinal cord lesion at T3 level seven years previously. On his re-admittance the deterioration of his function indicated that the lesion had risen to C7 level. As he was re-mobilized, he experienced severe pain in his left inguinal area, extending to the anterior thigh. There was some consternation when this pain persisted even after the cord was severed completely to relieve the pain.

On examination

There was no sensation in the legs and therefore it was not feasible to palpate for tenderness. These was normal sensation in the ears, however, and a tender area was found in the left ear which correlated to the hip joint.

Assessment

Although there was no motor or sensory sensation in the trunk and legs, the pain followed the stomach channel line and this was treated as a case of stuck *qi* in the stomach channel.

Treatment

First treatment: ST 29 (*guilai*), ST 36 (*zusanli*). A wooden chip was put on the tender point in the ear.

Second treatment: one day later, very little change. The same points were used.

Third treatment: one day later, had slept well and had been free of pain for 4 hours.

Fourth treatment: one day later, the same points on the ST meridian were used. In addition, a needle was put in the sympathetic point in the ear.

Fifth treatment: one day later, the same points were used.

Sixth treatment: following the weekend, there had been relief until Sunday afternoon and then the pain had returned.

Treatments were continued throughout the period of rehabilitation until discharge. The pain was not totally eased but the reduction in discomfort enabled the passive movement and exercise programme to be progressed.

Comment

This case is interesting in that there was no nerve supply to the trunk and legs and yet severe burning pain had been experienced. The needles were put in denervated areas and it was not possible to get *deqi*. The normal physiological pain relieving mechanisms giving short and long-term relief of pain could not have been stimulated. The pain probably originated in the sympathetic/ parasympathetic system and the needles had affected this part of the nervous system, about which comparatively little is known at present.

15.2.8 Sciatic/low back pain

Mr D., aged 48: This man was referred with left sciatic pain and low backache. He was an engineer involved in general duties.

History

There had been 5 years of intermittent pain which had been gradual in onset. It was worse in the afternoon and after any long period of standing or sitting. In the last 6 months it had been accompanied by severe spasm-like pains in the rectum which were very unpleasant. The latter symptoms were not associated with bowel motions and examination had shown that there was no sign of haemorrhoids. The spasms did however coincide with stressful situations. He also felt constantly tired yet could not get a good night's sleep.

On examination

Spinal movements were full range with some discomfort on over-pressure in extension and right side flexion. There was tenderness of lumbar 4 and 5 vertebrae on the left and in the area of the coccyx.

Assessment

In this case there was stuck energy (*qi*) in *du mai* which was also affecting the *yang qi* and in particular the bladder meridian. The tense personality and sleeplessness were all indicative of an excess *yang* condition.

Treatment

First treatment: BL 24 (*qihaishu*), BL 40 (*weizhong*); GV 1 (*changqiang*). Needles were left *in situ* for 20 minutes. Ear point *shenmen*: wood chip acupressure.

Second treatment: one week later. There had been improvement in the sciatica and no actual rectal spasms, but the preliminary tension prior to the spasms was still present. There was still disturbance of sleep. The same points were treated plus LI 4 (*hegu*) and LR 3 (*taichong*) to promote a better overall balance in body energies and to move *qi*. The wood chips in the ear were renewed.

Third treatment: one week later. There had been no pain experienced and he was sleeping through the night. The rectal spasms had now stopped. The wood chips in the ear were renewed and the patient asked to return in one week for a reassessment. No further treatment was given.

Fourth treatment: one week later. There was no pain in the back, leg or rectum. Spinal movements were full and pain-free. The patient was discharged. He returned three months later with a mild recurrence of the rectal spasm. A further treatment was given: GV 1 (*changqiang*) and GV 4 (*mingmen*). There was no further recurrence of pain.

15.3 CONCLUSIONS

Pain is a necessary physiological warning of dysfunction. Endeavouring to relieve pain without first diagnosing the cause could prove dangerous if it is a symptom of serious pathology.

Knowledge of TCM enables the practitioner to give a more effective treatment and it is possible to use acupoints on the opposite side of the site of pain with good effect. Phantom limb pain is one such condition which responds well to being treated as if the pain was on the intact leg/arm.

Many different techniques can be incorporated to treat the acupoints. These include TENS, laser, electro-stimulation and auricular therapy.

16

Headaches

16.1 INTRODUCTION

Traditional Chinese diagnosis of headaches is quite different from that of Western medicine. In TCM the circulation of *qi*, stagnation of blood and balance of *yin* and *yang qi* all have to be taken into account. The nature of the perverse energy which is the exciting cause of these disorders is also a factor in deciding on a treatment programme.

There are three diagnostic approaches that need to be addressed:

1. The underlying energic imbalances caused by external perverse energies.
2. The underlying energic imbalances caused by internal perverse energies.
3. The location of the pain relevant to the energic influence of the meridians in the area.

16.2 HEADACHES CAUSED BY EXTERNAL PERVERSE INFLUENCES

These are usually the result of invasion of Wind which may be combined with cold, heat or damp. They tend to be sudden and severe in onset, probably following exposure to draught or damp conditions. Being able to differentiate the cause of pain can give speedy resolution.

16.2.1 Wind combined with cold

This is sudden in onset, with pain radiating from the neck to the upper back. The patient dislikes wind and keeps the head covered. The symptoms are manifested in this way because the *yang* meridians meet at the head and are the first to be affected. The outer protective layer of the Six *Chaios*, *tai yang* (BL and SI), is affected, hence the pain distibution to the neck and upper back. The tongue will have a white fur and the pulse will feel as if it is floating.

Point selection
Points are chosen to disperse Wind and expel Cold, and could include a selection of local and distal points as follows: LI 4 (*hegu*), GB 20 (*fengchi*), GB 21 (*jiangjing*), GV 20 (*bahui*), TE 5 (*waiguan*), BL 12 (*fengmen*).

16.2.2 Wind combined with heat

This gives rise to a distended feeling in the head combined with severe pain, red eyes, flushed face, thirst, constipation and dark urine. The tongue in this case will have a thin yellow coat and the pulse will still feel as if it is floating but it will be rapid as well.

Point selection
Points should be selected specifically for eliminating Wind and Heat. These might include a selection of local and distal points from the following: LI 11 (*quchi*), LI 4 (*hegu*), GV 14 (*dahui*), GV 16 (*fengfu*), GB 20 (*fengchi*).

16.2.3 Wind combined with damp

The head feels as if it is in a tight band, the limbs feel heavy and weak. There is poor appetite, dizziness and drowsiness. There may be loose stools and difficulty in urination. The tongue will have a white greasy coat and the pulse a slippery or weak-floating feel.

Point selection
Points to expel Wind and Damp could include a selection of local and distal points from the following: LI 4 (*hegu*), ST 40 (*fenglong*), SP 6 (*sanyinjiao*), SP 9 (*yinlinguan*), GV 20 (*bahui*), GB 20 (*fengchi*), LU 7 (*lieque*).

If the perverse energy remains in the meridians for a period of time, the symptoms will become chronic and *qi* will be weakened. The periods between attacks will be pain-free but the headache will be initiated by changes in the weather and may be accompanied by nausea. Pain may start on one side of the head and spread over the whole head.

Treatment should include similar points to those described above but the needles should be retained for 15–20 minutes to supply the points and replenish *qi* energy in the meridians.

16.3 HEADACHES CAUSED BY INTERNAL PERVERSE INFLUENCES

The main diagnostic difference between these headaches and those initiated by external influences is the gradual onset of symptoms described. The actual pain experienced can be related to:

i. A *xu* (empty) condition when the pain will be dull and intermittent. Often the headache is not the primary cause of the patient seeking help, but is discovered on taking a case history, as part of a generalized *xu* condition.
ii. A *shi* (full) condition on the other hand produces severe headache and it is this condition which is met frequently as a primary reason for referral in practice.

16.3.1 Liver Fire headache

Symptoms will include: Intense throbbing unilateral pain, centred on the temple or behind the eye. The symptoms of Heat will be present, i.e. constipation, thirst, a bitter taste in the mouth, irritability, disturbed sleep. The tongue will be red and dry with a yellow coating and the pulse full, wiry and rapid. There will be the added symptom of nausea and vomiting if the stomach is also invaded by Liver Fire.

Point selection
The aim is to sooth the 'Fire'. A selection of the following points can be effective: LR 2 (*xingjian*), LR 3 (*taichong*), GB 20 (*fengchi*), GB 40 (*qiushu*). If there are stomach symptoms: ST 43 (*xiangu*), ST 44 (*neiting*), PC 6 (*neiguan*).

16.3.2 Liver *yang* rising – migraine

If the Liver Fire condition is allowed to become chronic it can lead to damage of the *yin* energy and a liver *yang* rising disorder will be the result. The symptoms experienced by the patient are those of a typical migraine (Blackwell, 1991). Chinese diagnosis further classifies the migraine according to the diagnostic features presented in the tongue pulse and other bodily signs. This analysis of the presenting pain enables treatment to be specific and effective.

(a) Liver blood xu

In this case the patient may experience spots and flashes in front of the eyes; photophobia, blurred vision, numb limbs and sallow complexion. The tongue will be pale especially at the sides, and the pulses will be thin and choppy.

(b) Liver yin xu

This is differentiated by the appearance of the tongue, which will be bright red with no coating, and the pulse, which is thin and wiry.

(c) Liver and kidney xu

In this case the main features are dry eyes and low back soreness, constipation and night sweats. The tongue will appear red with no coating and the pulse will be thin and rapid.

(d) Liver qi *stagnation*

In this case the pain is usual temporal and can either be unilateral or bilateral. The pain is felt as a throbbing distending pain and can radiate into the neck.

In women it may come immediately prior to the menses. It may well be brought on by strong emotional frustration or stress. The tongue may appear pale purple with small purple dots on the sides. The pulse will be wiry.

Point selection
All aspects of liver *yang* rising syndromes should be addressed in a treatment programme.

1. The weakened *yin* should be nourished using e.g. KI 3 (*taixi*), SP 6 (*sanyinjiao*).

2. The rising *yang* should be soothed using e.g. LR 3 (*taichong*), LR 8 (*ququan*). The paired organ GB will also be relevant, e.g. GB 20 (*fengchi*), GB 38 (*yangfu*). GB 41 (*foot linqi*) and TE 5 (*waiguan*) are the key points of *yang wei mai* and *dai mai*, the pair of the eight extra meridians concerned with the balance of *qi* in the upper and lower areas of the body and are concerned with the menstrual cycle.

3. Tension, which is often also a feature of liver-rising *yang* headaches, can be manifested following a period of stress when the patient begins to relax. The *qi* rises unrestrained and a headache results. Other points to ease tension or calm the *shen* (spirit) could be HT 7 (*shenmen*), PC 6 (*neiguan*), LI 4 (*hegu*), LR 3 (*taichong*).

4. Eye symptoms can be alleviated by using Extra point, *yingtang*.

16.3.3 Damp-Phlegm headache

The head swims, there is nausea and there can be vomiting of phlegmy saliva. The chest feels as if it is under pressure. The tongue will have a white greasy coating and the pulse will be slippery. The cause of this type of headache could be that of poor diet. Excess of fatty and sweet foods can lead to weakening spleen *qi* and affect its function allowing the internal generation of phlegm-damp. This then obstructs the passage of clear *yang* to the head.

This type of headache can be combined with liver *yang* rising, in which case the symptoms are intermittent. If a headache is treated as liver *yang* rising and is not responding to treatment it is worth considering that there is a Damp-Phlegm component even if the symptoms of this are not clear cut (Blackwell, 1991).

Point selection
Should be designed to eliminate damp, transform phlegm and replenish *yin qi*. A selection of the following points can be used: ST 40 (*fenglong*), a specific point to eliminate damp; SP 6 (*sanyinjiao*), the meeting point of the three *yin* channels of the leg; SP 4 (*gongsun*), the *lo* point of spleen; BL 20 (*pishu*), which is the *shu* point of the spleen; *yingtang* (Extra point) local to the pain. PC 6 (*neiguan*) and CV 12 (*zhongwan*) to alleviate nausea. ST 36 (*zusanli*) for stimulating the circulation of *qi*. LI 11 (*quchi*) for eliminating heat-phlegm.

16.3.4 *Qi* and blood *xu*

Pain is dull, prolonged and can affect the whole head. It can also be marked by pronounced dizziness and is better when the patient lies down, worse following over-exertion. There is a general malaise including loss of appetite, lack of concentration and physical weakness. The pain may begin at the eyebrows and radiate to the top of the head. There may be palpitation and heart flutters. The tongue will be pale with a thin coating and the pulses will feel thin and weak.

Point selection
This is designed to replenish *qi* and blood. A selection of the following points can be used: BL 18 (*ganshu*), the *shu* point of the liver; BL 20 (*pishu*), the *shu* point of the spleen; BL 23 (*shenshu*), the *shu* point of the kidney. Also ST 36 (*zusanli*), SP 6 (*sanyijiao*), CV 4 (*guanyuan*) and CV 6 (*qihai*) to replenish *yin qi*; LR 8 (*ququan*) to replenish blood; LR 3 (*taichong*), the *yuan* point of the liver; GV 20 (*bahui*), the meeting point of all the meridians and PC 6 (*neiguan*).

16.3.5 Kidney *xu* headache

The feature of this condition is the empty pain accompanied by dizziness. The pain may be at the occiput or the vertex and there may be soreness of the lower back. There can also be tinnitus and insomnia. The tongue will be very pale and the pulses thin.

Kidney yang xu

In this case the patient fears cold and there is a lack of warmth in all four limbs. The tongue will be pale and the pulses deep and thin.

Point selection
The aim is to nourish kidney *yin* and *yang* where indicated. A selection of the following points can be used: KI 3 (*taixi*) the *yuan* point; BL 23 (*shenshu*), LU 7 (*lieque*) and KI 6 (*zhaohai*); GV 4 (*mingmen*) to stimulate *yang*; GV 20 (*bahui*), CV 4 (*guanyuan*).

16.3.6 Stagnant blood headache

The nature of the pain is piercing and stabbing. It does not move around the head as in the other headaches. It is long-standing and continuous. It can be the result of trauma or the end result of the other types of headache described above.

Point selection
It is important to select points that will

1. Stimulate the movement of blood and *qi*, e.g. CV 6 (*qihai*) to move *qi*; SP 10 (*xuehai*) to move blood; BL 17 (*geshu*), SP 6 (*sanyinjiao*) and local and distal channel points.
2. Give local pain relief by using *ah shi* points.

16.4 THE LOCATION OF PAIN RELEVANT TO THE ENERGIC INFLUENCE OF THE MERIDIANS IN THE AREA (Figure 16.1)

The area affected by pain gives a clue to the meridians which are affected by perverse energy relevant to the Six *Chiaos*, i.e.

- The occipital area radiating to the back of the head and into the neck and upper thoracic spine is that area influenced by *tai yang* (BL and SI). This *Chiao* is most vulnerable to Wind-Cold.

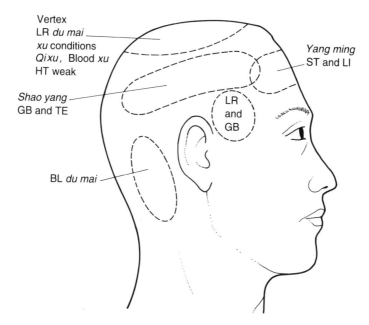

Figure 16.1 Headache syndrome areas. The site of the headache indicates a problem in specific meridians.

- The forehead and eyebrows, *yang ming* (ST and LI). This is most vulnerable to Wind-Damp.
- The side of the head radiating to the ear, *chao yang* (TE and GB). This is most vulnerable to Wind-Heat and can also be manifested by pain which starts at GB 14 (*yangbai*).
- The area of the Vertex and sometimes eyes and eyebrows, *tsui yin* (LR and HC). This can be affected by liver *yang* rising (Scott, 1984).

Point selection
Points which are listed below should be selected and used in conjunction with those described above affecting the *zang/fu*.

- *Tai yang* channels: BL 60 (*kunlun*), GV 14 (*dazhui*), SI 3 (*houxi*), BL 10 (*tianzhu*), BL 11 (*dashu*).
- *Yang ming* channels: LI 4 (*hegu*), ST 44 (*neiting*), ST 8 (*touwei*), GB 14 (*yangbai*), ST 36 (*zusanli*), *yingtang*.
- *Chao yang* channels: GB 41 (*foot linqi*) and TE 5 (*weiguan*); GB 20 (*fengchi*), *taiyang* (Extra) and local GB points on the head.
- *Tsui yin* channels: LR 3 (*taichong*), LR 2 (*xingjian*) to draw liver *qi* downwards. GV 20 (*bahui*), GB 2 (*tinghui*) local point, SI 3 *houxi*, which is the key point of *yang wei mai*.

16.5 DIAGNOSIS

Taking into account all the above information to form a diagnosis is a daunting prospect. Finding out when the pain is worse during 24 hours can give an important clue to the nature of the headache.

16.5.1 Time of day

(a) Worse in the morning

Qi and blood *xu* (*xu* type): This can give pain on waking and worsen during the morning.

Stagnation of liver *qi* (*shi* type): In this case the circulation of *qi* slows during rest and is often worse when the patient has overslept. Damp-Phlegm (*shi* type): Patients will often have a muzzy heavy head with swelling around the eyes.

(b) Worse in the afternoon

This is the *yang* time of day and *yang* type headaches due to full or empty heat are likely to be more severe at this time, i.e. liver *yang* rising and liver fire and kidney *yin xu*. Those involving *liver qi* stagnation which are due mainly to stress can be exacerbated as tension rises during the day.

(c) Worse in the evening

These are usually *xu* type headaches. The pain increases as the patient becomes more tired.

16.5.2 The effect of the weather

(a) Worse in hot weather

Retained Wind-Heat, kidney *yin xu* or liver fire.

(b) Worse in cold

Retained Wind-Cold, blood stagnation or kidney *yang xu*.

(c) Worse in damp weather

Retained Wind-Damp or internal Damp-Phlegm.

(d) Worse in changes of weather

Retained external pathogenic factor or liver *qi* stagnation.

16.5.3 The effect of the menses

If the pain is worse immediately before the period then the cause is stagnation of *qi*.
If it is worse during the period it is due to stagnation of blood.
If it is worse after the period, it is due to a blood *xu* condition.

16.5.4 The effect of exercise

Exercise exacerbates pain when there is a *xu* condition causing the headache.

In the case of liver *qi* stagnation the pain is often relieved by exercise although it will return when the patient rests.

16.5.5 The effect of palpation/massage

If there is hypersensitivity this indicates a *shi* condition. Where there is relief on deep pressure, this indicates a *xu* condition. Massage is beneficial in both cases although it is initially very uncomfortable in the former. It stimulates *qi* and blood and has a dispersing effect on the *shi* headache and a stimulating effect on the *xu* condition.

16.6 TREATMENT

When pain is acute distal points only should be stimulated and if there is no relief after 5–10 minutes local points can be added. Between headaches distal points can be used on their own. If there is a *shi* condition then a 'reducing' treatment is used, if a *xu* condition a 'supplying' technique is necessary.

Mobilizing techniques on the cervical spine where indicated and postural correction and advice on working/resting positions are an essential part of the treatment programme.

Headaches experienced on waking may be exacerbated by sleeping in an incorrect position. This can often be remedied by advising the use of a butterfly pillow. This is a simple device where the top pillow (it must be a feather one), is tied in the middle thus pushing the feathers to each side to form a butterfly shape. The narrow central part is where the neck is placed and the 'wings' act as a splint to prevent involuntary tossing and turning during sleep. If the patient turns onto the side, the extra bulk of the pillow fills the gap created between the point of the shoulder and head, thus maintaining a reasonable postural position.

16.7 DIET

Headaches are often affected by food and drink. It is useful to know the effects of various substances on the body in TCM terms. For example:

- Alcohol: In Western terms it is a substance that can have a damaging effect on the liver. In TCM terms it generates

Damp-Heat. The Heat affects the liver and the Damp weakens the spleen function to generate Damp-Phlegm. It has a dispersing effect on *qi*, pushing it upwards towards the head and can thus trigger a Liver Fire headache.

- Tea and coffee: These both contain caffeine. In Western terms this drug inhibits the midbrain in its function of responding to painful stimuli. The result is that there is more pain experienced. In TCM terms tea and coffee have a similar effect to alcohol in that they disperse *qi* upwards and outwards and also deplete *yin* and blood.
- Red meats and fried food: These are classified as Hot and Damp. They can aggravate Liver Fire or *yang* rising.
- Dairy products: These generate Damp and Phlegm.
- Citrus fruits: These are considered to be Cold and to weaken the spleen, thus Damp-Phlegm is generated. The extra dampness may then aggravate liver *qi* stagnation.
- Sugar: Has a weakening effect on the spleen and thus generates Damp.
- Chocolate: Generates Damp-Heat, The Heat affecting the liver and Damp the spleen.

Advice on diet is an important part of the treatment programme. If the underlying cause of the dysfunction is a particular food then the treatment will only be partly successful if the irritant is not identified and withdrawn from the diet.

Thus, if a patient has a headache which is diagnosed as having a Damp-Phlegm component for example, those foods which generate this condition should be withdrawn from the diet.

16.8 CASE STUDIES

16.8.1 Migraine A

Mrs A., age 42.

History

This lady complained of migraine once a week for 14 years. It had started after the birth of her third child. Pain was always on the left side of the head in the temple area and in this year had increased in intensity. She had had a stressful summer and had felt very irritated all the time. She had developed a taste for sour foods. She had been to a migraine clinic where a prescription containing ergot had been given, which had relieved the pain. She was on no medication, at the time.

On examination

She gave the impression of being tense and anxious. Movement of the cervical spine were restricted in left rotation and in right side flexion. There was tenderness at 2nd cervical apophyseal joint left. Pulses felt wiry and there was weakness in the Water pulses and fullness in the Wood pulses. Tongue was pale, wide and had toothmarks along the sides.

Assessment

This was a liver *yang* rising headache.

Treatment

First treatment: LI 4 (*hegu*), LR 3 (*taichong*), GB 20 (*fengchi*), KI 3 (*taixi*). Mobilization C2 level grade 11/left rotation and right side flexion were clear.

Second treatment, one week later: Movement of cervical spine was clear. There had been no further change in symptoms. The tongue and pulses were unaltered. She had had a migraine two days previously. LI 4 (*hegu*), LR 3 (*taichong*), TE 5 (*waiguan*) and GB 41 (*zulinqi*): these are the key points of *dai mai* and *yang wei mai*. SP 6 (*sanyijiao*).

Third treatment, one week later: She had had a migraine but it was not so severe as previously. On examination there was improved colour in the tongue. There was still weakness felt in the KI pulse. The points above were repeated.

Treatment continued for a further six weeks, at the end of which time there was definite improvement in general well-being and there had been no migraine for two weeks. The patient was discharged.

16.8.2 Migraine B

Mrs P., age 50.

History

This very small, tense lady had suffered from migraines since chidhood. No treatment had helped. They could last from 1 day to 1 week and were severely disabling. The GP referring felt that there was a strong precipitating emotional factor in this case. The pain did not favour the right or left side of the head.

On examination

There was no notable joint problem. Pulses weak on the right wrist and stronger on the left wrist. Tongue small and red with white covering fur.

Treatment

First treatment: In view of the history I felt that this problem was a profound internal one brought about by some allergy to food. I discussed this with the patient and she agreed to go on an elimination diet. I also spoke with her medical practitioner to check that there was no contraindication to this course of action. The patient was warned that if my diagnosis was correct, she would experience a severe headache within 48 hours as this would be a withdrawal response of the body to the exclusion of the allergenic food. No acupuncture was given.

Second treatment: There had been a severe headache (worse than ever) two days following the commencement of the diet but nothing since. She also felt better. She was advised to add in one item of food per meal, leaving bread to the last, as this takes longer to go through the digestive system and can cause symptoms 24 hours after ingestion.

Third treatment, one week later: There was no return of pain. The patient phoned after a further week and said that on drinking coffee for the first time she had experienced a severe headache, otherwise all the other foods that had been added had been taken without ill effect.

The nine food diet

The patient can eat any of the following but cannot have any seasoning, and must drink bottled water: lamb, cod, trout, parsnips, turnips, carrots, courgettes, celery, pears.

NB This case illustrates the importance of diet in some long-standing problems which are met in clinical practice.

16.8.3 Occipital pain

Mrs T., age 46.
This lady had occipital pain which had started while away on holiday 6 months previously. There was no particular pattern to the headaches and general health otherwise was good. The last 10 days she had felt off balance when moving around.

On examination

Cervical movement: all clear except right rotation which was reduced by 25%. Tongue: pink and scalloped at the edges. Pulses: floating.

Assessment
This appeared to be a headache due to external perverse Wind affecting *tai yang*.

Treatment

Points to dispel Wind affecting *tai yang* were chosen and exercises to improve neck posture were shown. GB 20 (*fengchi*), GB 34 (*yanglingquan*), BL 10 (*tianzhu*), GV 14 (*dazhui*) GV 16 (*fengfu*).
Second treatment, one week later: Very much better, but still some residual pain in the occiput. The treatment was repeated. After a further two treatments the symptoms were resolved.

16.9 CONCLUSIONS

Treatment of headaches/migraine is a good illustration of the importance of the environment on the body. Meticulous assessment as to whether the condition arises from external or internal pathogenic influences is essential for a lasting successful outcome. Advice on diet, lifestyle and mobilizing/manipulative techniques all form a part of a treatment programme.
Headaches which are sudden in onset and appear to have no notable history should be treated with caution and full investiga-

tions to exclude serious pathology should be advised before treatment is attempted.

REFERENCES

Blackwell, R. (1991) The treatment of headache and migraine by acupuncture. *Journal of Chinese Medicine*, Number 35, Jan., 20–26.
Scott, J. (1984) Diagnosis and treatment of headaches by acupuncture. *Journal of Chinese Medicine*, Number 15, May, 5–20.

Other conditions which are met in clinical practice

17.1 INTRODUCTION

Acupuncture is part of a complete system of medicine and any disorder can be addressed using the TCM concepts of treatment.

Some conditions are more efficiently resolved when treated in the Western way. Others can be treated with a combination of Western and traditional medicine.

The disorders addressed in this chapter are those that are most likely to come within the remit of physiotherapy practice.

Important treatment note: Treatment using acupuncture for any presenting condition when the patient is pregnant or is hoping to become pregnant must be approached bearing in mind that certain acupoints are contraindicated at this time. These are: SP 6 (*sanyinjiao*), LI 4 (*hegu*) and abdominal points throughout pregnancy. Also all points below the umbilicus in the first five months (Low, 1990).

17.2 OBSTETRICS AND GYNAECOLOGY

The uterus is considered in traditional Chinese texts to be one of the extraordinary organs of the body. It is governed mainly by ancestral energy and the meridians most involved with its function are:

- Triple Energizer: with its ancestral energy connection.
- *Ren mai* which controls the *yin* meridians and has particular relevance to the uterus.
- *Chong mai*: the 'sea of blood' which originates in the uterus and controls the supply of blood to the pelvic area and regulates the *qi* and blood in the 12 main meridians.

- *Yin chiao mai*: assists removal of stagnent *qi* and blood from the lower abdomen and is involved in the function of the genitalia.
- *Dai mai*: controls the balance of *qi* in the upper and lower abdomen.
- Kidney: is the source and store of ancestral energy and nourishes the uterus.
- Liver: governs the flow of *qi* with *ren mai*. It helps to store blood with *chong mai* and with the spleen it helps to keep blood in the blood vessels. The LR meridian supplies the area of the Fallopian tubes.
- Spleen: holds the blood in the vessels and supports the pelvic viscera (Low, 1990).

17.2.1 Diagnosis

Factors which have to be taken into account in gynaecological problems:

- The influential meridians.
- The balance of *yin* and *yang qi*.
- Whether it is a full/empty condition.
- Whether it is a hot/cold condition.
- Whether it is stagnant *qi*, blood or *yin*.

17.2.2 Morning sickness

Treatment for morning sickness with acupuncture is often requested, as the taking of anti-emetic drugs is prohibited during pregnancy. There is some difference of opinion amongst practitioners of acupuncture as to the safety of using needles during the first three months of pregnancy. The points listed below can all be stimulated using acupressure treatment.

- PC 6 (*neiguan*), specific for vomiting.
- ST 36 (*zusanli*), the *ho* point of the stomach.
- LR 2 (*xingjian*), the Fire point of the liver channel.
- ST 40 (*fenglong*), to eliminate Damp-Phlegm which can cause acid regurgitation.
- CV 12 (*zhongwan*), local stomach point.

NB Ear acupuncture is contraindicated in the first five months of pregnany and after five months the acupuncture points of uterus, ovary, internal secretion, abdomen and pelvis cavum should not be needled, as premature labour can be the result (Huang, 1975).

17.2.3 Pain during labour

In China acupuncture is sometimes used as an anaesthetic for Caesarian sections but not routinely as an analgesic.

It can be very effective in reducing pain in the first stage of labour and can be used to reinforce uterine contractions in the second stage. In clinical practice the practitioner must be prepared to attend the patient at any time when labour commences. This entails obvious practical difficulties in rearranging appointments for other patients.

Treatment

Attendance in the labour ward can only be a successful procedure when the full cooperation of the midwife and medical practitioner is obtained.

TENS is widely used in Western medicine. The careful placing of the electrodes on acupuncture points should enhance the analgesic effect. It is helpful if the patient can practise using the stimulator in the final weeks of pregnancy so that she is fully acquainted with the sensation it gives and the control of the intensity, etc. The electrodes can be placed over BL 23 (*shenmen*). This will stimulate *qi* to the kidney and BL 24 (*dachanshu*) local for lumbar pain. Special obstetric TENS, which have a basic frequency of 2–15 Hz, are used to stimulate the midbrain to give long-term pain relief and also have a burst mode of high frequency at 100–150 Hz giving a more immediate effect during the contractions.

Acupuncture can be added to this treatment in the following ways.

First stage

The purpose is to promote relaxation and reduce pain, while supplying the organs to enable the uterus to function efficiently in its preparation for parturition. Points used are GV 20 (*bahui*) and LI 4 (*hegu*): this is a strong analgesic point and is specific for back pain. It also stimulates the movement of *qi* and strengthens contractions. LR 3 (*taichong*) to calm the liver and also to promote the circulation of *qi*. GB 34 (*yanglinguan*) which together with *hegu* and *taichong* helps to move and balance *qi* in the whole body.

Second stage
This can be speeded if indicated by supplying LI 4 (*hegu*) and either SP 6 (*sanyinjiao*), the meeting point of the three leg *yin* meridians (LR, SP, KI), all of which are important in the function of parturition, or ST 36 (*zusanli*) to stimulate *qi*.

17.2.4 Premenstrual tension

This is often met in practice because of the associated pain and discomfort experienced in this disorder. A careful case history should indicate whether pain or emotional disturbance is due to a disorder in the monthly cycle. It can present as a headache. This has been addressed in Chapter 16. It can also present as fatigue combined with oedema of the legs. In this case the cause is probably kidney and spleen *xu*.
Treatment could include:

* BL 20 (*pishu*), the *shu* point of the spleen;
* BL 23 (*shenshu*), the *shu* point of the kidney;
* GV 4 (*mingmen*), to reinforce the kidney;
* CV 4 (*guanyuan*), specific for the uterus;
* ST 36 (*zusanli*), influential point for stimulating *qi* in the meridian system.

Another symptom is often that of depression or extreme irritation. These are both symptoms of liver disorder, the former due to liver *qi* stagnation which can then give rise to the latter, rising liver fire. Treatment will aim to move the *qi*.
Treatment could include:

* BL 18 (*ganshu*), the liver *shu* point;
* BL 19 (*danshu*), the gall bladder *shu* point;
* LR 3 (*taichong*), the source point of the liver;
* LR 14 (*qimen*), the front *mu* point of the liver.
* SP 6 (*sanyinjiao*), to move *qi* in the three *yin* meridians of the leg.
* GB 41 (foot *linqi*), to open *dai mai*.
* If there is breast pain, KI 3 (*taixi*) to stimulate *yin qi* in the kidney.

17.2.5 Dysmenorrhoea

This painful condition has two main aetiologies:

1. It can affect girls from the time of their first period through to childbearing, when the problem is resolved. The cause of the disorder is not clear but may be due to hormonal disturbance.
2. It can affect older women who previously have had no pain. In this case there is usually an organic reason for the problem and this needs to be identified before treatment is started. Close liaison with the patient's medical practitioner is important.

Treatment

This will be depend on the nature of the symptoms.

Local points could include: CV 3 (*zhongji*), CV 4 (*guanyan*), CV 6 (*qihai*), CV 12 (*zhongwan*), BL 32 (*ciliao*), BL 29 (*zhonglushu*).

Distal points: GV 20 (*bahui*), SP 6 (*sanyinjiao*).

PC 6 (*neiguan*) for nausea, LI 4 (*hegu*) specific for pain.

If there is stagnation of *yin*, the pain is usually felt centrally and there is often diarrhoea or constipation. Massage and heat relieve the pain. Points are selected to move the *yin*, e.g. CV 4 (*guanyuan*) moxa, SP 6 (*sanyinjiao*), SP 10 (*xuehai*) specific for heat in the blood, BL 23 (*shenshu*) to move *yang*.

If there is a full *yang* condition there is pain on pressure usually on the left, with some relief with cold. The pain is spasmodic. In this case the *yin* should be stimulated by supplying SP 6 (*sanyinjiao*) and the *yang* drawn upwards by treating GV 20 (*bahui*) and local bladder or abdominal points.

If there is fullness of *yin*, pain is worse on pressure, usually on the right side of the pelvis and is better with warmth. There are spasmodic pains appearing before the menses.

Treatment should be aimed at balancing *yang* and *yin* by moving *yin* and supplying *yang*: CV 4 (*guanyuan*) to get *yin* moving and ST 40 (*fenglong*) which sends the *yang* energy from the exterior the interior.

If there is stagnation of blood, the symptoms are of severe stabbing pain occurring at the onset of the menses. It may radiate to the thighs and low back. Treatment should be directed to regulating blood and *qi*:

CV 3 (*zhongji*) specific for the uterus and the Lower Energizer;

CV 6 (*qihai*) to move *qi*;
SP 10 (*xuchai*) specific for blood;
SP 6 (*sanyinjiao*);
SP 4 (*gongsun*) to open *chong mai* (Low, 1990).

The treatment for dysmenorrhoea should ideally be given a week prior to the onset of the menses and repeated at monthly intervals over the next 4 to 5 months. Acupuncture treatment can be combined with massage, heat and exercises for the abdominal muscles and swimming is also an excellent way to mobilize *qi*.

17.3 URINARY DISORDERS

According to TCM these disorders arise as a result of imbalance in the following meridians: CV, SP, KI and GV, ST, BL.

The organ which is the most significant is the kidney. In Chinese medicine this is not only the organ itself and its function but includes the adrenal glands, testes and ovaries.

17.3.1 Nocturia

This is a condition which is frequently a problem, particularly for elderly people. It is not usual for this to be a primary source of referral but is often a distressing symptom for those who have arthritic disease.

In Western terms it could be hypothesized that acupuncture affects the detrusor muscle of the bladder through the sympathetic/parasympathetic nervous system. In TCM urinary disorders are the result of a disorder of kidney *qi*.

Treatment

The main point to use is SP 6 (*sanyinjiao*). This balances the *yin* and *yang qi* of the kidney and also supports the abdominal viscera. ST 36 (*zusanli*) stimulates *qi* in the meridian system.

17.3.2 Stress incontinence

This can be the result of pelvic floor weakness and/or uterine prolapse.

The standard physical treatment for this disorder is to teach pelvic floor exercises and in some cases stimulate with faradism (this works through the motor points of the voluntary muscle to stimulate pelvic floor contractions). Training with weighted cones is also effective in many cases.

There are some patients, however, who do not respond to this treatment and interferential treatment has proved very helpful. This is applied using a sweeping frequency of 10–100 Hz. This stimulates both the voluntary muscle through the motor nerves and the smooth muscle through the sympathetic nervous system. It is interesting that the electrodes are often placed on the inside of the thigh and on the left and right of the abdomen and it is through these areas that the kidney and spleen meridians pass. Stress incontinence is very often the result of uterine prolapse. This is the result of a *xu* condition in TCM terms. Electrical stimulation of the kidney and spleen points which lie under the interferential electrodes are affecting the *qi* in the kidney and spleen. Stimulation should not be prolonged as this will cause 'sedation' of the points and exacerbate the *xu* condition. The optimum time is 15 minutes which takes into account the sweeping frequency used.

The *qi* can be reinforced by treating

- SP 6 (*sanyinjiao*);
- CV 3 (*zhongi*) Moxa;
- CV 4 (*guanyuan*) Moxa;
- GV 20 (*bahui*) is added to draw energy upward in any prolapse condition of the pelvis.

NB Acupuncture and electrical stimulation are only effective in early prolapse. If the patient presents soon enough surgery can be avoided in many cases.

17.4 HEMIPARESIS

This is treated widely in China. According to TCM this condition results when there is an invasion of Wind. Therefore the GB meridian is significant. This perverse energy penetrates to the *yang ming* layer of the Six *Chiaos* which is formed by LI and ST. Thus the points on these three meridians are primarily used.

The treatment is aimed at moving *qi* and blood and eliminating Wind (in TCM terms). In Western terms the reduction of muscle spasm and restoration of coordinated function is the aim.

The points listed below are those that are found to be most effective. Selection will depend on the pattern and severity of the paralysis. It is important to remember that muscle spasm is a result of insufficient *qi*. Supplying GB 34 *yanglingquan* is always a good idea as part of the treatment formula as it is the influential point for muscle. The patient will probably be generally weakened and the use of moxa giving energy in the form of heat can be beneficial.

The acupuncture treatment should relieve some of the muscle imbalance and thus facilitate re-education of function. The method of physical rehabilitation is a matter of choice for the practitioner but could include Bobath, Peto, Rood and PNF techniques. Acupuncture can be incorperoted in all these modalities.

17.4.1 Hemiparesis affecting the arms

(a) Local

LI 15 *jianyu*, LI 11 *quchi*, LI 4 *hegu*, EX 28 *baxie*, TE *jianliao*, TE 5 *waiguan*, TE 3 *zhongzhu*.

(b) Distal

GB 34 *yanglinguan*.

17.4.2 Hemiparesis of the leg

(a) Local

ST 32 femur *futu*, ST 36 *zusanli*, ST 37 *shangjuxu*, ST 40 *fenglong*, ST 41 *jiexi*, ST 44 *neiting*, EX 36 *bafeng*, GB 34 *yanglinguan*, GB 37 *guangming*, GB 40 *qiuxu*.

(b) Moxa

CV 6 *qihai*, CV 4 *guanyuan*, BL 23 *shenshu*, BL 25 *dachangshu*, LI 11 *quchi*, SP 6 *sanyinjiao*, ST 36 *zusanli*, ST 41 *jiexi*.

It is difficult to evaluate the efficacy of acupuncture on hemiparesis. It is certainly worth pursuing as a preparation for other physical rehabilitation.

17.5 MYALGIC ENCEPHALOMYELITIS
(ME, POST-VIRAL SYNDROME)

This is a condition that is increasingly met in clinical practice. The symptoms can arise following severe viral infections. One cause of this condition can be identified as an invasion of Wind which is not fully expelled from the body. The remaining pathogenic factor stays in the interior as Heat or Damp-Heat. This affects the body in two ways. It weakens the resistance to external perverse influences and the Damp-Heat inhibits the function of the stomach and spleen, which further weakens the interior. Thus, a vicious cycle is set up (Maciocia, 1991). The disorder manifests itself as either an Excess or Deficient condition. Some are described below.

17.5.1 Excess conditions

(a) Damp-Heat in the muscles

Signs and symptoms
Fatigue, aching muscles, lack of concentration and muzziness. Tongue: sticky yellow coating. Pulse: slippery.

Suggested points to eliminate Damp-Heat
SP 9 *yinlinguan*, SP 6 *sanyinjiao*, SP 3 *taibai*, BL 22 *sanjiaoshu*: all effective for eliminating dampness; LI 11 *quchi* to eliminate Damp-Heat, CV 9 *shuifen* and CV 12 *zhongwan* for the transformation of body fluids, thus helping to resolve Damp. Points should be treated evenly or sedated.

(b) Heat in the interior

Signs and symptoms
Muscle fatigue without pain, thirst, insomnia, breathlessness, cough with scanty yellow sputum and loss in weight. Tongue: red with a yellow coating. Pulse: rapid and wiry.

These symptoms usually arise in the early months of the disorder and then convert to the Damp-Heat syndromes.

Suggested points to clear interior Heat

- GV 14 *dazhui* to clear long standing Heat.

- TE 5 *waiguan*, LI 11 *quchi* to eliminate Heat.
- SP 6 *sanyinjiao* nourishes *yin* which helps to cool Heat.

17.5.2 Deficient conditions

(a) qi *deficiency*

Signs and symptoms
Fatigue worse at the start of the day, lack of vital energy, shortness of breath, sweating during the day, poor appetite and loose stools. Tongue: pale. Pulse: empty.

Suggested points to tonify *qi* and expel remaining pathogenic factors

- ST 36 *zusanli*, SP 6 *sanyinjiao*, BL 20 *pishu*, BL 21 *weishu*: all to tonify ST and SP;
- CV 6 *qihai*, for general tonification of *yin*;
- BL 13 *weishu* to tonify lung *qi*.

These points can be supplied with Moxa unless there is residual Heat.

(b) Yin *deficiency*

Signs and symptoms will vary according to which organ is affected. The most likely ones to be affected are the lung, stomach, spleen and kidney.

(i) Lung
There will be exhaustion, dry cough, night sweating, breathlessness. Tongue: red without coating or with coating only at the front. Pulse: floating/empty.

Suggested points to nourish lung *yin* and *qi* are LU 9 *taiyuan*, CV 17 *shanzhong*, BL 13 *feishu*, DU 12 *shenshu*, CV 12 *zhongwan*, ST 36 *zusanli*, SP 6 *sanyinjiao*. All **not** to be supplied with Moxa.

(ii) Stomach
Signs and symptoms are fatigue, dry mouth, epigastric pain, dry stools, malar flush. Tongue: normal colour with midline crack or transverse cracks at the side. No coating in the centre. Pulse: general feel fine and rapid, but the ST pulse floating/empty.

Suggested points to nourish *yin* and strengthen ST and SP *qi* are: ST 36 *zusanli*, SP 6 *sanyinjiao*, CV 12 *zhongwan*, ST 44 *neiting*. Supply the points.

(iii) Kidney
Signs and symptoms are: soreness of lower back, exhaustion, weak legs and knees, tinnitus, deafness, insomnia, night sweating, dryness of the mouth. Tongue red without coating. Pulse: floating-empty or rapid-fine.

Suggested points to nourish *ki yin* and strengthen the kidneys are: KI 3 *taixi*, *yuan* point of kidney; LU 7 *lieque* and KI 6 *zhaohai*; CV 4 *guanyuan*, SP 6 *sanyinjiao*, BL 23 *shanshu*. Supply the points.

17.5.3. Conclusions

As the practitioner becomes familiar with the signs relating to deficiency and excess and the peculiarities associated with individual organ dysfunction, further syndromes can be worked out. Treatment of ME requires a great deal of patience from both the patient and practitioner.

17.6 CASE STUDIES

17.6.1 Early uterine prolapse

Mrs J., age 34, referred by GP with early prolapse of the uterus.

History

Patient had prolonged labour with first child and developed an intermittent 'bearing down' sensation following parturition. There was no stress incontinence.

Two years later she had a second child; the symptoms were more marked and the baby was 8 months old. There was still no stress incontinence. On examination the pelvic floor muscles were of normal strength. There were no particular changes to remark on in either the tongue or pulse.

Treatment

SP 6 (*sanyinjiao*), ST 36 (*zusanli*), CV 4 (*guanyuan*). All needles retained 20 minutes (supplying).

Second visit, one week later: There had been a temporary relief of symptoms lasting 48 hours. Treatment was repeated using above points plus GV 20 (*bahui*).

Third visit, one week later: Symptoms were much improved. Treatment was repeated.

Fourth visit, three weeks later: Symptoms had all returned after 5 days without acupuncture. Treatment was changed to interferential to pelvic floor combined with GV 20 (*bahui*).

Fifth visit, one week later: Very much better and effect had lasted through to present visit. Treatment was repeated, combining interferential and GV 20 (*bahui*).

Sixth visit, symptoms almost resolved.

After three further treatments the patient was discharged.

17.6.2 Myalgic encephalomyelitis

Mrs H., aged 28.

History

Developed ME following severe thoat infection and several courses of antibiotics. She presented with severe pain centred in her neck and low back. She was unable to walk more than a few paces and lived a virtual wheelchair life.

On examination

She was very overweight and had a pale bloated look. Tongue was bright red without coating.

Assessment

This was a kidney *yin* deficiency.

Treatment

She was treated with local points for the pain in the neck and shoulders and systemic points, i.e. KI 3 *taixi*, KI 6 *zhaohai*, SP 6 *sanyinjiao*.

There was slow recovery and increased stamina, but it took two courses of treatment over one year to achieve this. Treatment was combined with exercise within the patient's tolerance.

REFERENCES

Huang, L.H. (1975) Rules against acupuncture treatment, in *Ear Acupuncture: The Complete Text* by the Nanking Army Ear Acupuncture Team, Rodale Press Inc., Emmens, Pennsylvania.

Low, R. (1990a) Acupuncture physiology, in *Acupuncture in Gynaecology and Obstetrics*, Thorsons Publishers Ltd, Wellingborough, UK.

Low, R. (1990b) Disorders of pregnancy, in *Acupuncture in Gynaecology and Obstetrics*, Thorsons Publishers Ltd, Wellingborough, UK.

Maciocia, G. (1991) Myalgic Encephalomyelitis. *Journal of Chinese Medicine*, Number 35, Jan. 5–19.

Index

Betablockers, Chinese pulses and
140
BI syndromes 224–5
Biao, see External disorders (*biao*)
BL (urinary bladder)
acupoints, *see* BL (urinary
bladder) points
Five Elements theory 10, 11, 12
meridian theory 27, 70–80
command points 34, 35–7
distinct meridians 45
energy flow 30, 31
long *lo* meridians 42
transverse *lo* meridians 39
Six *Chiaos* and 21, 22
see also Fu organs; Water
element
BL (urinary bladder) points
73–80
BL 1 *jingming* 45, 73, 161, 163
BL 2 *zanzhu* 73
BL 3 *meichong* 73
BL 10 *tianzhu* 25, 45, 73–4, 227,
272, 278
BL 11 *dashu* 25, 74, 162, 272
BL 12 *fengmen* 74, 266
BL 13 *feishu* 74–5, 155, 159–60
allergies 247
asthma 244, 245, 246
bronchitis 74, 248
myalgic encephalomyelitis
289
post-operative chest
disorders 249
BL 14 *jueyinshu* 75
BL 15 *xinshu* 75
BL 16 *dushu* 75
BL 17 *geshu* 75, 162, 224, 227,
271
BL 18 *ganshu* 75, 270, 283
BL 19 *danshu* 75–6, 283
BL 20 *pishu* 76
asthma 245
bronchitis 248
headaches 269, 270
myalgic encephalomyelitis
289
premenstrual tension 283
BL 21 *weishu* 76, 289

BL 22 *sanjiashu* 76, 288
BL 23 *shenshu* 76–7, 227
asthma 246
back pain 154, 261
BI syndromes 224
dysmenorrhoea 284
headaches 270
hemiparesis of leg 287
joint disorders 76, 223
myalgic encephalomyelitis
289, 290
premenstrual tension 283
BL 24 *quiashu* 77, 231, 261, 263
BL 25 *dachanshu* 77, 282, 287
BL 26 *guanyanshu* 77
BL 27 *xiochangshu* 77
BL 28 *pangguangshu* 77
BL 32 *ciliao* 77–8, 284
BL 39 *weiyang* 78, 234, 239
BL 40 *weizhong* 78, 161, 162,
228, 234, 263
BL 55 *heyang* 78
BL 57 *chengshan* 78
BL 58 *feiyang* 42, 78
BL 60 *kunlun* 78–9, 234, 272
BL 62 *shenmai* 79, 110, 116–17,
162, 234
BL 63 *jinmen* 79
BL 65 *shugu* 79
BL 66 *tonggu* 79
BL 67 *zhiyin* 79–80, 164
Blood
headaches and 270–1
sea of meridians/blood 25, 26
Blood disorders 75
circulatory 50, 66, 88, 164, 188
hyper/hypotension 52, 92
Bones, *see* Musculo-skeletal
problems
Bronchitis, acupoints 59, 70, 74,
248–9

Cardiac disorders
acupoints 66, 106
angina pectoris 64, 66, 75,
83
palpitations 83, 106
tachycardia 83
yin wei mai 114, 115